BUCK!

BUCK!

EVERY-CRICHTON

Buck the Menopause

Buck!

Published by Buck the Menopause in the United Kingdom 2023
Tel: +44 (0) 7596 762524
Tel: +44 (0) 7960 876007

This is a work of fiction. Any similarity between the characters and
situations within its pages and places or persons living or dead is un-
intentional and coincidental.

Book design by Deidre Crichton and Susanne Every
Jacket Design by Deidre Crichton and Susanne Every
Jacket photograph based on the work by sculpture artist Matt Buckley
Image courtesy of justsculptures.com/products/edge-sculpture-venetian-carnival-mask-teal

First Printing, June 2023
Printed and bound in Great Britain by IngramSpark.

To our family and friends. It's finally here!

Foreword

Buck what?

- Buck the trend?
- Buck the midlife crisis?
- Buck the menopause?
- Buck the stereotypes?

Yes, that's it, all of the above.

How does this book work?

You'll meet six women who tell their life stories until now. They are different characters from different backgrounds with various dilemmas. What they have in common is that they're all in their middle years and 'change' is happening.

With menopause a hot topic currently, these women, consciously or not, are all tuning in to a series of digital media in the form of podcasts, short videos and weblogs. These digital media segments are relevant to their stories. They contain information pertinent to help them, and you, the reader. So slow down and absorb. Like them, you will gain an awareness because every chapter offers valuable insights.

The seventh character, narrator of her own story, will reveal herself as the book unfolds. And, of course, the eighth character is YOU.

This book is a work of fiction; however, the information in the media segments is factual and well-researched. Note to family and friends. You will not find yourself. Every character is at least a blend of three people: the known, the known of and even some deceased.

| 1 |

What lies behind the mask?
(They see/She feels)

I'm Jane, your hostess. Some of you will know me from my former life as a journalist, others from my books, *I am a woman, not a small man* and *Where is happy Granny?* For a few of you, it will be from my more recent charity work with *Complex, supporting women around the globe*, hence the recent honours, but I remain humble, curious, and … post-menopausal.

This podcast is the first in a series of digital media forms to explore the challenges of a woman's midlife. This period (pun intended), or stage of our lives, is when our shifting hormones bring new comforts and concerns, along with a few interesting and sometimes unwelcome physical and mental changes.

Each podcast will either enlighten, educate or entertain. Make no mistake; we will delve into the good, the bad, and the downright ... ty. Let's face it, if *we* don't talk about these issues, who will?

Some topics, by their very nature, will be serious, if not heavy, but ... team and I will endeavour to keep it light and find the humour wherever possible. Believe me, the future looks bright. But first, let's uncover some layers.

All of us wear masks at some point in our lives. They can be a simple face covering for protection or elaborately decorated for theatre to disguise or conceal. Now think about the symbolic masks that we wear. Even the face of bravado is its own mask presenting confidence over uncertainty. The poker face is a blank mask designed to be clueless. Consider these masks as we start this series with a 'feary tale' of Queen (Cinder) Ella as she approaches her fiftieth birthday. King Charming is planning a grand masked ball to celebrate, and Ella is about to make her biggest mistake. She wishes for her fairy godmother to complete her Menopause Journey in just 24 hours.

Be careful what you wish for.

This tale is not for the faint-hearted; grab a chair, turn on the fan, and … let's begin.

Once upon a time

There lived a most gracious and beautiful Queen, Ella, who was admired and loved throughout the kingdom. Although she had endured a very shaky start in life (her beloved Mother, then Father had died), she met and married a Prince, who became King. Together they live happily ever - now, raising their many children to adulthood and making sure the whole kingdom thrives.

Lately, Queen Ella's older not-so-attractive step-siblings were getting her down. Hour by hour, day after day, and week after week, she had listened to the moans and groans of their tales of menopause.

Surely menopause could not be that bad, she thought.

She knew that 'Woeful' and 'Really Woeful' were prone to exaggeration and attention seeking, but they painted a very grim picture.

So when her Fairy Godmother called by to grant Ella her 50th birth-day wish, Ella asked that her menopausal journey be fast-tracked and completed within twenty-four hours. "You know, get it over and done with and through to the other side," she reasoned.

The fairy godmother warned that this was a bad idea, but Ella was adamant, so reluctantly, the fairy godmother agreed to grant Ella's wish.

"The spell will start at midnight on the eve of your fiftieth birthday and end 24 hours later as the clock strikes twelve midnight. There will be many new experiences, my dear, and you can only break the spell by going to the fountain of youth in the courtyard and chanting three times:

*'**Peri**-sh the **meno, post**-haste.'*

If you don't chant the phrase in time before the clock strikes twelve, all the changes will remain and become permanent. Good luck, my dear."

"Don't worry, Fairy Godmother, I'll take a fan to overcome those hot flushes I've heard so much about," she said casually.

The Fairy godmother casts her eyes to heaven, and then she casts the spell.

Poof!

*Our story begins at **1am** as Ella is having night sweats. She thinks she's in a nightmare as she blows hot and cold. She'd flung pillows and duvets about the room; her nightdress was soaked. She feels sticky and gross. Charming is getting really pissed off as she's interrupting his beauty sleep. She must have fallen asleep again but awakes at **3am**, in the witching hour, desperate to go to the loo. Tinkle over, Ella returns to bed but cannot settle. Her brain's engaged, and all senses are on high alert; is the clock ticking too loudly, or is Charming breathing too deeply? Anxious thoughts start building and grow into catastrophic thinking. At **5am**, at last, she falls asleep.*

6am, the alarm goes off. She turns over and sees the glint in Charming's eye. "Not now, darling, just a little cuddle; I promise to bump uglies later." She says reassuringly.

Ella feels that her boobs are a bit tender. At 7am, she curses in the shower as she realises her hair needs washing again. Then, with shock, she spots a stray grey pubic hair in her patch.

Never mind, it's a busy day with charity events and a meeting with the engineers working on the moat. "I need to be taken seriously."

Ella chooses a pinstripe corset with hooks and laces in the back. She glances backwards in the mirror to check her silhouette but is slightly alarmed.

Good grief, my arse looks big! She thinks. Anyway, focus.

She takes a second to smooth her locks and quickly plucks a pesky, wiry grey hair that appears to defy gravity. It's spoiling her groomed look. Once harvested, she's ready to start the day.

It's 9am, and as she's walking through the palace, she receives an admiring glance from a dashing footman and has a fanny flutter. Still got it, she thinks comfortingly.

At 10am, she's in a meeting with the engineers and builders and is alarmed when she loses her thread of thought. Take a second, breathe. Now back to the conversation, especially regarding points on her checklist. Just as she recovers from that, she feels a heat surge starting. Suddenly she has overwhelming panic and is preoccupied with the heat and possible redness of her face and neck—first the flash, then the flush. I'm out of control, she thinks, mopping her brow. She's forgotten the damn fan, but even so, she wouldn't use it as it would only draw attention, and she would lose her credibility.

By **10.30am**, her corset suddenly feels tight, and she surreptitiously loosens the bow at the back for comfort. However, she can hear the ping, ping, ping as the hooks release the laces, and she's left with the very real threat of the corset unravelling. She summons her trusted servant, Buttons to save the day by adjusting and relacing her corset.

At **11am**, her coffee has left her with a metallic aftertaste, and she wonders if they've used Civet poo beans again. She's very cross because the eco-warrior in her made it abundantly clear that this was unsustainable, and she had banned it throughout the kingdom.

11.30am, as patron of the new children's home, she attends an opening ceremony, where she must give a speech and reveal a plaque behind the red velvet curtain. While there, she squats on a tiny stool to read a tale to the children, but to her horror, she feels the tell-tale whoosh, followed by warm wetness. It's an unexpected period. And a heavy one. Buttons spots the crimson flood and quickly rips off the velvet curtain, drapes it around her middle, helps her to her feet, and announces, "This will make a lovely skirt for you, madam." She moves off, much to the disapproval of the onlookers who suspect that the queen may already have quite enough red velvet in her possession.

By **12.30pm**, Ella is cleaned up, padded up, and good to go again. She realises that her next engagement is at the other end of the park, and together with her entourage, they decide to walk the journey. Admiring the horse chestnut trees, she stoops down to collect the conkers used to deter the spiders in her room. She's oomphing and aahing with every pickup but is unaware. So when Buttons offers to collect these for her, it's surprising when she quickly responds, "Sod off, Buttons."

In the park, they enjoy the sunshine and the ducks paddling in the lake. Buttons produces a bag of bread pieces to feed the ducks and offers it to Ella. She smiles as she accepts, but after a while, she turns to her group and notices their faces showing alarm.

"What?"

"I thought you would gently feed the ducks, Ma'am, not take aim and fire at them," Replies Buttons.

1pm, at the orangery, lunch is a medley of buffet delights, and she can't wait to indulge. Ella realises that she's hungry, actually starving. With only one opportunity to fill her plate, she does just that. Buttons marvels at this teetering tower of delicacies and is already on- guard to catch this precariously balanced smorgasbord, which she duly devours. But she's not done. Ella still craves something sweet and insists that there is room for puddings. Having once been a moderate drinker, Buttons is now amazed at how many glasses of wine she's managed to neck over lunch.

At **2pm**, Ella leaves in her carriage with her ladies in waiting. She has a bout of acid reflux, and her stomach begins its orchestral sounds. Bloating causes stomach pain, and it wants soothing. The only way is out. She uses the poor suspension of the carriage to gently roll from side to side and release the gas slowly. Not sure where it's going, as it's not coming out the usual way. Delighted that there is no smell in the carriage, she assumes that the vapours must be hiding in the folds of her dress.

3pm, they arrive back at the palace, and as she stands up to leave the carriage, the longest and completely uncontrollable queef or fanny fart lets rip and startles both the horses and her entourage. She doesn't notice the awkward glances and titters of her staff. The horses continue whinnying, so she's reassured. She got away with it.

3.30pm Ella's dressmakers call to deliver her ballgown, but she is struggling to remember the names of this design team. It's only been two days since they were last here. "Oh, what are their bloody names?" she mutters but is quickly appeased. The dress is beautiful, and she's delighted. Yet minutes later, she's in a foul mood, with no idea why.

4pm Her eyes feel scratchy and dry. Maybe her contacts need to come out. They have simply got to go as she frantically blinks to moisten them. But where has she put her reading glasses?

4:30pm Ella is in the library corresponding with one of her children. Her heart starts pounding like it's jumping out of her chest. Terrified, she raises the alarm, but the palpitations have stopped by the time Buttons arrives. Panic over. She continues her correspondence, only stopping to pull out a reference book. The dust cloud that follows the book's withdrawal starts a bout of sneezing.

"Uh oh." Sneeze, pee, sneeze, pee. Despite clenching with all her might, Ella cannot stop the spurts. "Damn it!" Knicker reinforcements are needed again.

5pm: It's time for a light supper. Ella asks Cook to prepare a handful of quail's eggs with celery salt and some asparagus with hollandaise. She insists on having a double gin and tonic because it's happy hour too. Charming makes his appearance, sees the large, now empty glass and thinks he's in with a chance of having a quickie. He flashes a twinkling smile and pulls her into her dressing room. Ella is not interested; there is still so much to do. It doesn't matter how much Charming kisses and fondles; her drawbridge stays firmly shut. He persists, and with a bit of sweet talk, she's softening. Wielding his battering ram, he makes steady progress but is soon met with physical resistance. Finally, the portcullis slams shut. Damn. Charming stomps off grumpily; he knows when it's time to retreat.

6pm Ella showers and rewashes her hair. The clumps that come away in her hand are now primarily grey. Thank goodness she's wearing a wig tonight. As she soaps her nethers, she notices her pubic patch looks like a sodding iron-grey steel wool patch. It feels like it, too, a sparse one at that. While towel drying, she contemplates which body butter best serves her crepey skin. While bending down to cream her legs, she feels the start of another hot flush. "Goodness's sake, I'm drenched; into the shower I go again." Finally, the dress goes on, and she's shocked as it's too tight. Two days ago, it fitted like a glove; now she's muffin topping. Her ample curves are spilling out everywhere, her back, her waist, even her groin area. Another flush announces itself as she's finally strapped into the dress. The burnt orange silk is now flambéed in dark orange wet patches. She likes her wig, but as they place it on her head, it weighs heavily, and the after-flush causes rivulets of sweat to run down her neck. A headache has started brewing. "Great!" Intelligently, she swops her famous glass slippers with their dainty high heels for platform trainers. They prove to be far more comfortable on her swollen cankles.

Finally, at **7pm**, wig and mask firmly on, Ella and Charming make their way to the front of the palace entrance as their Ball guests start to arrive. As hosts, they have to greet everyone in the line, but it was taking too long, far too long. As the guests trickle through the doors, she feels a personal trickle developing. Charming leans over and discretely whispers, "You're fidgeting; what's wrong with you?" Before she can reply, she desperately needs to pivot and bolt fast, in three, two, one ...

At **8pm**, the gong sounds the call to dinner. Ella realises she can't read the menu; she's forgotten the damn glasses again. Before taking a seat, she nips to the library and, having found said glasses, again tries to read the menu. "Damn it," they don't work anymore. She searches for the magnifying glass and sees her reflection in the window. She notices that her face looks orange, starkly contrasting her pale turkey neck. Her eyebrows are no longer visible as they have thinned and gone grey. Her eyes have sunk and appear smaller and dull. Her jawline is less defined. Her lips are thinner and feathered. Her teeth have become putty coloured. She looks stressed, as stressed as she feels. Also so unbelievably tired. Gratefully she puts the mask back on and sets out to join the dinner guests.

At **10pm** the after-dinner talks begin. As the speeches take place in the hushed hall, she's aware that she's in excruciating pain from her gut activity and the build-up of trapped air. Slow release means that the silent but deadly gasses come thick and fast. Around their circular table, guests have started flaring and twitching their nostrils. The microclimate she has now created around her makes her a social pariah. The servers have stopped attending their table, and Charming is getting more than pissed off as their glasses need recharging for the toasting session.

At **10.30pm** the dancing begins. As Ella takes to the floor with her charming husband, she notices how pale her hand is in his, and it is now covered in age spots. Her knuckles look knobbly, and her nails are brittle and broken.

As the couple sway, her new bingo wings sway to their own tune. She knows the wet patches under her arms are on show and worries that the clear zone around them is to do more with her odour than royal etiquette. But she needn't be concerned; these new pheromones are turning Charming on, and along with the mystique of the wig and mask, his loins are well and truly stirred.

11.30pm He is determined to have another go and whizzes her around the room towards the exit, finding a quiet spot on the terrace, where he once again tries to seduce his wife with whispers of sweet nothings in her rather long-lobed ear. Slow, gentle and loving is what Ella wants, but Charming's efforts are paying off, and she ardently returns his kisses with her ever more thinned lips. The moonlight reveals her putty-coloured teeth, and startled, he pulls away. But determined to seduce his wife, Charming puts this glimpse down to a trick of the light. He feels the rough whiskers on her chin. She fears they may be rivalling his. As he releases her corset, he tries to grab her breast but finds they've dropped significantly, and the nipples now point at her feet. So he decides to spin her around and enter her from the rear. Cinders shouts, "Ouch, ouch, that's painful!"

Charming, desperate now, needs finishing off. He spins her back again and gently pushes Ella onto her knees, positioning her head firmly near his groin area. Enthusiastically, Ella wants this too, but her knees are killing her, a flush is imminent, and the mask keeps getting in the way. Just then ...

The clock starts to strike. **DONG**. Startled by the sound, her head turns quickly, causing the wig to come away in Charming's hands. **DONG**. He looks down and sees a strange old lady about to fellate him, and his ardour rapidly deflates. **DONG**. She painfully staggers from her knees to her feet, and he pulls the mask away. **DONG**. "Who are you?" he shrieks. At that exact moment, the terrace doors are flung open as guests spill out for the fireworks display **DONG**. She moves away from him and starts heading towards the fountain. "Wait, Ella, you've been bewitched," he calls in pursuit as he eventually recognises her. **DONG**. Guests become obstacles in her way to the fountain. "Move!" she screeches as she bashes a champagne glass out of the hands of a guest, and it shatters, parting everyone in its wake, **DONG**.

The courtiers see an old lady, an intruder, being chased by Charming, and they try to intercept her. **DONG** They shout, "Wait up, old lady," as they continue to give chase. **DONG** She grabs a silver tray from a serving boy, and wielding it like a machete, she bashes a way through anyone in her path. **DONG** Buttons comes towards her, "F*** off, don't even think about it! she growls. **DONG** Looking ahead, she can see the plume of the three-tiered fountain drop a level. Now she has a clear way forward. Another plume drops. With every ounce of her being, she sprints to the fountain (the crowd sees an old lady hobbling, oomphing and gasping), and then she sinks to her knees at the water's edge.

"**Peri**-sh the **Meno**, **Post**-haste,

Peri-sh the **Meno**, **Post**-haste,

Peri-sh the **Meno**, **Post**-haste."

It's midnight. **DONG**

The final water plume drops.

Nothing happens.

Ella bows her head in defeat as it appears that's she too late.

After 10 seconds of silence, the gurgling noises begin, and the rushing water surges up as the fountain of youth is restored to its former glory, and so too is she.

Charming rushes to his wife's side and says, "Darling, you're back; where have you been?"

Quietly she sighs, "**You don't know the half of it.**"

THE END

The moral of this tale, apart from 'being careful what you wish for,' is that menopause, like pregnancy, is about making gradual adjustments and, of course, awareness, monitoring, and information.

While this tale was a bit of fun, the reality is that we should all know ahead of time which hormonal stage we're in and what it could entail. Searches online are so scattered. Without a joined-up approach, this information is almost impossible to navigate. Which gives the message of trial and error or suck it and see.

This feary tale of the thirty-four most common menopausal symptoms was a rollercoaster for poor Ella.

Did you spot them all? Did you determine which symptoms were mental and physical and which can damage the spirit?

In truth, we rarely experience all these symptoms; we have our collection. Even then, you may share the same list with a friend but still have a hugely different rhythm. Moreover, all symptoms differ in frequency and intensity.

We may hear that ¾'s of women experience hot flushes. But how many per hour, per day, or even per week? What about duration? For how long? Think how many seconds, how many minutes?

What about sex and libido? On the one hand, eighty per cent of women report vaginal dryness, and that low libido is common. But on the other hand, we have anecdotal reports of the over-sixties confirming that they are having their best, most fulfilled sex life ever.

It's all so random. Lots of information. Who are you listening to? What's your source? Statistics or anecdotes?

So if women have been on the planet since the dawn of time and we now represent fifty per cent of the population, surely there has to be a guide that will prepare us for what is to come in menopause. There is. The most relevant tool is 'The menopause rating scale' (MRS).

This scale fills the gap, as before 1990, there were no standard-ised scales for measuring the intensity of our symptoms and their corresponding impact on our health and quality of life.

It's easy to complete and freely available online. The link is in the notes.

It's a self-efficacy rating questionnaire. The eleven questions have a scale of 1-4. And the sub-scores for each category: your head (Psychological), your body (Somatic), or your nether regions (Uro-genital or Sexual) helps you to explore your discomfort levels.

The total score can indicate how big a deal this stage of your life is, ranging from no or negligible complaints, to mild, moderate, or severe. The questionnaire is a good starting point for any conversation with a medical professional. It's a gauge for a moment in time. However, time changes, and so too does the score. So you will need to keep revisiting your discomfort levels.

Numerous studies have shown that you're more likely to suffer from symptoms like night sweats and anxiety during your perimenopausal stage. In addition, while vaginal dryness and incontinence are more likely to start in menopause, they can also build during post-menopause. It all sounds rather grim, but it is not a given eventuality.

There is help at hand and options every step of the way.

Maybe you don't want to even acknowledge some of these symptoms yourself, never mind draw attention to them with others. But all sorts of remedies are out there. Be prepared to be lonely and scared if your only friend and confidante is an internet search engine.

And, of course, as your menopausal journey unfurls, so does your ageing body's progression. The two are intertwined. We're all just moving targets. What will you attribute to hormones, and what represents ageing? Hand in hand, your general health and this hormonal shift will determine what choices are available to you.

Along with knowing your medical history, your general practitioner will assess your symptoms according to the Straw+10 study and is likely to suggest that you do a blood test that will indicate your hormonal levels at a point in time. Natural menopause is confirmed when twelve months have passed since the last menstrual period. The global average age of menopause is fifty-one. (1996 WHO)

This assessment will enable you to review your options and determine what suits you.

Prescribed treatments for the symptoms escalate as follows:

- Lifestyle changes
- Nutrition and exercise
- Natural remedies and supplements
- The medical route, such as HRT
- Or combinations of the above

Time to get even more serious. Ok, so the natural menopausal age may be fifty-one, but we all know various friends and family who are early or late. What else can fast-track these symptoms?

Other causes are:

- Genetics (what was your mother's age?)
- Autoimmune diseases
- Infections
- Medical-related triggers, such as hysterectomies, oophorectomy (ovary removal)
- Radio and chemotherapy treatment
- Smoking
- Poor eating habits
- Caffeine
- Alcohol
- Sleep deprivation
- and other combinations of known or unknown factors

These are all checklists that inform the professionals. Yet, at an individual level, it's far more complex. The bottom line is that all women will follow their individual journey. We all have our backstories and events that have shaped our lives. These events, good and bad, have affected our physical and mental health. How we arrive at menopause will shape our narrative going forward. Following the lessons learned, you can prepare for all eventualities, review all options and select the most relevant ones wisely.

In a nutshell, successfully managing this stage of our lives begins with **Awareness** of where you're at, **Finding** the information or help, and **Selecting** the best options available.

You will want to tune into my next podcast. What can I say? It's bound to be tantalising.

And don't forget, we appreciate you sharing your stories and wish to continue to hear more real experiences from real women. We are all so amazingly complex.

Until next time. Stay cool.

| 2 |

Tamsin's story

"I'm going to pin my colours to the mast here; I'm thinking of leaving Steven. It's time to focus on this next stage of my life."

"What-the-fuck Tamsin. Why?" Julian asks, nearly choking on his latte.

We're sitting in our favourite coffee shop. It's where our working day begins. Julian works for the same IT company. I'm his boss, but if you asked, he'd say he is my right hand. Which is to say, *he* manages *me*. He is an indispensable member of the team and a confidant and ally I didn't think I'd ever need. I trust him implicitly. More than I trust Steven, I think. Julian seems to be able to read my mind daily. But, it turns out, he did not see this coming.

"So, pray tell," he says, dabbing at the foam spotting his Burberry coat, "just what has prompted this thought?"

Where do I even start? How do I even begin?

"I'll tell you what, Jules, let's save this discussion for another evening. I will spill the beans over a bottle or two of our favourite red. For now, tell me when my meeting with Richard is scheduled. Christ, we'll need to distract him today. I'm feeling rather out of sorts," I say, gathering my coat. "Let's get the hell out of here; another busy day awaits."

"Tamsin, wait up!" Julian rolls his eyes at the waitress. "God, she's incorrigible!" He catches the eye of the drop-dead gorgeous new barista and mouths, "Call me," as he drops a fiver upon which he's written his mobile number into the tip jar, and then rushes to catch up with me.

"If this is your idea of conversational foreplay, I can't wait for the climax. Right, your first meeting is at nine in the boardroom, briefing the app team, followed closely by a zoom call with our South African team. Oh, and Richard wants half an hour of your time at twelve. He'll be on the warpath about the deadlines on that AI driven 'smart health' app you're working on."

It's late afternoon. I'm back at my desk. I've endured a rather tricky morning. I feel the stirrings of what feels like period pain again. This is uncharacteristic. I'm not due to come on for another week. As I brush aside the thoughts of my reproductive system, I'm free to think about how my day began. Nothing unusual: the alarm buzzing, Steven reaching over to turn it off before I can get to it. He rolls back to face me and kisses me. Smooth move. It's a technique he's perfected over the years. This used to go one of two ways: either we'd go through the motions of practical lovemaking or jump out of bed and start the day in earnest. Today it was the latter. I follow him to our en suite, where he begins his morning rituals by splashing his face with cold water. He brushes his teeth while cleaning the area around his basin. He does this every morning in the same order. I watch him and wonder if he senses that I'm a different person today. Of course, he doesn't; I keep this mask firmly in place. He tries to catch and hold my eyes in the mirror above our separate washbasins. These tender glances used to give me such comfort.

Today I don't make eye contact. Instead, I stand there brushing my teeth, noticing how tidy his shelf is. Everything is clean and neatly stacked; he needs this order. Until now, I've never really noticed how much of a mess I leave in my wake, how he has always patiently restored order not just to his own space but to mine as well. Today this thought hits me in the ribcage, and I gasp.

"Alright?" He asks, looking concerned.

"Sure, just wind", I say, turning away while rubbing my chest. My heart feels fluttery and achy, and I'm unsure what this means. As I prepare to shower, Steven leaves to wake the twins. They will soon begin their morning routines. I hear their reluctant stirrings and his soothing reassurances. This family I didn't ask for and now cannot imagine life without. I've betrayed them all. The dutiful wife and loving mother masks sit uneasily today. I take extra care soaping myself as I remember what happened last night. I am bruised all the way down my back to my bottom. I stand so that the warm water runs down my back, and as I feel these tender spots awaken, my vagina contracts with recognition and longing for the cause thereof. My lover is responsible for this feeling. He promised me that he would leave no mark unless it was what I wanted. I wanted it badly. That's my only control – I can make him stop anytime. Last night I didn't want it to end.

We all meet later at the breakfast table, where I greet the children, check the family schedule for any involvement on my part, and wash down my daily supplements with a glass of orange juice. Then I prepare to leave. Steven ushers the children out the door and into the car, ready to drop me at the train station before setting off on the school run. This has been our morning routine for as long as I can remember. We spent most of our married life caring for these little people who defied all odds and were thrust quite unexpectedly into our lives.

I work in the city, holding a senior director's role in a technology firm, while Steven is a psychotherapist working for a local practice. Having trained and worked in mental health for most of his life, he now specialises in disorders such as depression, anxiety, and PTSD. The months following the pandemic changed the dynamic in the home drastically. As the demands on his time grew, so did the responsibilities around our family and home life. This past year has been a shitshow for all the obvious reasons but for us, the unrelenting schedule clashes. Though most occurred online, I've had to do more than my usual share of school-related activities and attend parent-teacher meetings. Steven's patient base grew, as did the time spent in lockdowns. This work-and-school-from-home dynamic played havoc with our home life and relationship as we juggled meetings, childcare, and all the domestic stuff that suddenly took on many layers of complexity. All this while working on one of the most significant projects of my career to date. When we both couldn't attend a series of parent-teacher meetings, compounded by our twins being in separate classes with varying learning challenges, it blew the lid off of what we knew was an already sizzling pressure cooker. We had our biggest row yet. I'd been telling him for months to employ an au pair. He promised to scale back his patients so that we'd have his time back. It didn't happen. HE LOST IT COMPLETELY when I mentioned boarding school for the twins.

"You care more about your meetings and work deadlines than about us. I know you're busy, but these are our children, and they need you to be involved in their lives, too," he yelled.

"Oh, I care, all right; I care that you all live in this comfortable home, that the children are in a good school, and that you never want for anything—all thanks to me. Don't tell me that I don't care," I shouted back.

"Tamsin, you can be so bloody insensitive sometimes. I'm not asking for much, a little help and support now and then. Instead, your response is to bring strangers into the house to raise our kids or ship them off to boarding school. Something we both agreed was off the cards."

"A little help and support? Are you fucking kidding me, Steven? I'm the main breadwinner in this house, and yet I'm expected to keep picking up the slack. Perhaps you should consider what else we agreed on at the start of this parenting path. It was never going to be about your career! I'll stay at home, you said. I'll take care of them, you promised."

"Can't you see how the world has changed, Tamsin? My skills are needed now more than ever! All we're doing is adapting to this new way of living. It will be good for us."

"Good for you, you mean!" I snarked.

Steven wouldn't budge, and neither would I. So, as with most of our disagreements. I left him to stew.

When the twins were born, he was pretty willing to be the main childminder and homemaker. This decision took little thought; it just happened. After a rather painful and traumatic birth, I could not breastfeed them, so with Steven quite adept at bottle feeding, I quickly resumed my job as head of software development. It never occurred to either of us for me to stay at home. The money was too good; besides, I didn't have the time, whereas his work was sporadic, plus he could work from home. It was an arrangement that suited us, and it worked. I needed the structure of my job and desperately needed to be with people. I thrived on the buzz in this ever-changing and dynamic industry. Soon the company became even more successful, and I was required to travel more frequently again, so I started meeting with our clients worldwide. Of course, there was the initial guilt, but I consoled myself with the fact that I was a significant role model for the twins. We both were; there would be no gender stereotyping for us, thank you. Increasingly, they became Steven's responsibility as they grew older, and he loved it. He was quietly confident and having them in his care around the clock didn't faze him. I was happy to acknowledge his primary parent role and ensure he was rewarded with special treats. These included tickets to all the international rugby matches, all at my company's expense – they were sponsors and had a hospitality suite at Twickenham. In the summer, front row seats to the tennis at Wimbledon. Perks of the job. Overall, it made for a happy and stable home. After my travels, it always felt good to return to this calm but sometimes messy house. To spend the last part of the evening snuggled up and reading to the twins. By then, Steven would have fed them, bathed them, and ensured they were ready for bed; delightful. That warm, comforting baby smell became my reset every evening. What a joy!

Steven became immensely popular at all the parent-toddler social and play classes and relished in the day-to-day minutia of the children's lives. Sometimes I felt resentful of the amount of time he had with them. Although on the more difficult days, and there were plenty of those, I was relieved to escape. I made sure to do my share of parenting on the weekends. If I didn't actively participate, it would result in the silent treatment. I'd be on the receiving end of that. This no-speak would sometimes last for days and make things awkward between us. The latest self-help book or a bestseller was always a good icebreaker. I'd have our office assistant order and deliver it to the house. Steven was a voracious reader in his spare time, so this was an instant get-out-of-jail-card for me. Dinner was the grown-up's time. He usually cooked, but I would collect something on the way home if the mood was fraught. His professional perspective on office politics and a decent bottle of red improved my day considerably. Which meant the sex was good. I liked mine fast, rough with some role-play, while he wanted the drawn-out foreplay and the post-sex pillow talk. We settled for somewhere in between. Over the years, we continued in much the same vein. As the twins became older, their routines changed accordingly, but our relationship remained unchanged. He gave all his time and energy, and I took it all.

So how did all this lead to my wanting to leave him? At last, I feel like the real me again. Finally, someone has thrown me a life buoy that stops me from drowning in this life of mediocrity. I am weary of the pretence of it all. I am tired of wearing the appropriate mask for each occasion and always making the necessary adjustments when it feels like it's slipping. I wonder if Steven feels the lack of spontaneity as I do. Our life, the sex, feels like I am being force-fed vanilla ice cream when all I want is to taste the variety of flavours in the cart. And boy, have I tasted them all!

I didn't want to marry Steven in the first place.

Our families were friends. Growing up, we lived in the same seaside town and belonged to the same sailing community. However, we were never close friends. We attended separate schools; but his friends were my friends, and vice versa. This network kept him on my periphery with the occasional chance encounter at the sailing club. I spent most weekends sailing or kayaking, practically living on the water in the summer months. In our early teens, occasionally, we'd find ourselves on the same vessel. A mutual admiration developed for our boating skills, and we soon were on the same team in competitions. Although I was slight, I was strong and earned my position on the boat. By eighteen, we were firm friends, and our families decided that we, as a couple, were perfectly matched. I was the feisty one, happy to show my true colours. I loved taking risks and always sought thrills by sailing close to the wind. Steven was quieter, more stable, and preferred to sail with an even keel. Our sailing temperaments seemed to spill over into our university lives. Different universities, thank God. My computer science degree was tough, but I coped with the stress of exams by partying hard. On home visits, my choice of the rugger bugger types was a source of amusement for everyone, Steven included. He joked that I was a sucker for punishment, as my type appeared to be The Jock – tall and attractive but could only talk rugby, even amongst this sailing crowd, and they were given stick for that. His girlfriend, another salty, whom he'd met in fresher's week and two years later was still seeing, was nice, pleasant even, but oh so very dull. I thought they were ideally suited.

I enjoyed our flirty exchanges. Our endless sailing chat meant we often huddled at family gatherings—nobody minded, not even our partners. Well, maybe his girlfriend seemed displeased, as she regularly ingratiated herself into our discussions. The families continued to tease us about being soulmates and we were often asked, "When will you make it official?" I continued to provoke him. I loved to hint at my sexual exploits. I could see how uncomfortable he felt to hear what I liked in bed. He was reading Psychology at university, and perhaps he was psycho-analysing my bad behaviour. He confessed that he felt intimidated by me. At parties, I'd wait for his girlfriend to turn away, catch his eye, and wink, while biting my lower lip suggestively. I knew how to turn him on. I danced slowly and seductively to show him and every man in the room what my body was capable of. It thrilled me to think that I would be on his mind when he was fucking her later.

Our families had been going to church together for years. As we went through these rituals, I wondered what other sacrifices were needed to find happiness. I considered how different I was from my parents. They'd married young and had never really left the confines of their community. Their livelihood and their contentment came from the familiar. Even my twin brother was settling. He was happy to live the life of our parents. Steven's parents were like that too. They shared similar morals and values, never giving in to temptations beyond the world they knew. He admired that, whereas it made me feel claustrophobic, and I couldn't wait to escape. I wanted more from life. I needed to maintain forward momentum, keep changing direction as required, and keep adjusting my sails to catch the wind. The thought of being in a committed relationship felt like a punishment and not a reward. Even our minister reminded me he'd be delighted to conduct our future nuptials. Talk about pressure! Anyway, Debbie, the dull-ightful girlfriend, looked like she would stay. His family liked her, and so did mine.

After my Masters, I joined an IT company in the city. This placement put me at a turning point in software development. I worked my way up through the ranks, and by the second year, I was directing a sizeable team. This new role involved international travel. We had satellite offices in big cities around the world. At first, it seemed coincidental that I'd strike up a conversation with a stranger in a hotel bar and then end up in bed with them. Soon I looked forward to when I could frequent clubs and bars at the end of a busy workday, on the prowl for my daily sexual fix. It was a game, really. Some nights I toyed with them for hours; other nights, I couldn't get them into my room fast enough. One shameless encounter led to us fucking on the stairwell up to my room. It was the allure of it, the thrill of being caught and knowing I could be anyone I chose to be in this city full of strangers. I wore many different guises, and I allowed each fantasy to play out to fruition.

By my late twenties, I was still unattached and happier for it. I was travelling frequently and indulging my appetite for the forbidden. My bedroom games now included a growing fantasy toolbox with leather restraints, clamps, and various spanking implements, each adding another layer of thrill. My hand luggage would sometimes get searched, and I'd receive either a wink and a knowing smile or silent disapproval. Usually, during these exploits, I'd be on the receiving end of pain – the submissive; however, occasionally, I'd meet someone, usually a powerful CEO type, who wanted to be dominated by me. I was always happy to oblige. To be handed that much control was exhilarating. I felt powerful, invincible. In those moments, I wasn't the only one wearing the mask. My justification? I worked exceptionally hard, so I enjoyed the rewards along the way. Monetary or otherwise. I was wonderfully comfortable and could afford to live well. In addition, I was very satisfied with my sex life. I had it all.

"I need you to meet with a big client in New York," said Richard, my boss. "I know you've just come back from South Africa, but this is urgent, and you know that I wouldn't ask unless it's important."

My flight was already booked; he knew I'd say yes, and so off I flew. Meeting over, business concluded, Richard happy, now for my reward. I felt jetlagged and somewhat jaded, but nothing that a stiff drink and some bedroom antics wouldn't cure. Maybe I was off my game that evening or feeling reckless, but the guy I chatted up and lured back to my room with the promise of tantalising fun was not my usual type. For one, he didn't bother to take off his wedding ring – they usually do, and another thing, his bloodshot eyes were a clue to his having taken something far more potent than alcohol.

Furthermore, he didn't play by the rules. His chokehold sent fear coursing through my body, real fear and not the exciting kind I expected. As I tried desperately to break free, I scratched him and drew blood. He took it as further encouragement and flipped me over while pinning my tethered wrists behind my head. His strength was terrifying, and I kicked and writhed in pain as he entered me from behind. He tore into me repeatedly. This form of punishment had no pleasure in it for either of us. His climax brought no relief to him; I sensed that. His erection never subsided. He entered me again, and this time the pounding was relentless. When he finally finished, he let me go, muttering, "You asked for that, you stupid bitch!"

I lay curled up in a ball as I watched him gather his things, dress and leave. Like an animal, I bit and tore at the leather restraints on my wrists to free myself. Only then did I allow myself to surrender.

I cried for two days, too hurt to leave the room, too weak to seek help. I made excuses for missing my flight and requested some time off work upon my return. When I finally returned to the country, I went straight to my parent's house, home. I couldn't talk about what had happened. They wouldn't understand. I blamed myself for my bad judgement. I knew that I'd been lucky thus far. It had only been a matter of time before the risks I took caught up. I told everyone I was exhausted, with too many business trips, long working hours, and a chronic lack of sleep. My body took a week to heal, but my mind took far longer. Finally, after a few weeks, I found the courage to look ahead and put the rape behind me. I told no one.

A few months later, I bumped into Steven in London. We were grabbing takeout meals from a favourite restaurant. He looked good. Sad, but good. I knew from my parents that he was newly single and that Debbie had broken his heart. Call it fate, pity sex, or rebound sex. Whatever it was, we ended up having it, and it felt safe, it felt tender, and it felt familiar. We parted the next morning. Two months later, I found myself in A&E having to have a routine pregnancy test; It was a positive result. The scan confirmed it— two heartbeats, loud and clear. Abortion wasn't an option for me, being a twin myself. It was time to chart a different course. Steven needed to be involved. He insisted on attending subsequent scans with me; a boy and a girl they revealed, an instant family. To say we were shocked initially was an understatement. I'd always been so careful with birth control. My proclivities, the rape, a chance meeting, and our one-night stand; all led to this very moment. There was only one possible outcome when we shared the news with the families—a hastily arranged marriage. Steven and I were swept up in a whirlwind of planning and preparations until the day finally arrived sooner than we would have liked. We expressed our doubts, and everyone else was pleased. The night before the wedding, I called him.

"Steven, you know we don't have to go through with this, right? It feels like an arranged marriage. I feel ambushed."

"I know, but we both know the alternative is far worse. We'd also be letting down many people," he stated.

"I'm financially comfortable; I can do this by myself. It's easy to employ people."

"What's my role to be then? An occasional daddy? I want to be there for them every step of the way and be there for you too. I know you, Tamsin, this will be good for us. Everyone agrees," he offered.

"You don't know me at all. You only know the Tamsin from the past. I'm different now."

"I've known you my whole life. Please think of this as a fresh start for us. Trust me, this will work out," he promised.

The wedding went ahead as planned, apart from a slight glitch, on my way down the aisle. I'd paused, hesitant as I faced the sea of expectant faces. It was only the look of certainty on Steven's face that gave me momentum. Ultimately, thankfully, the events on that day went swimmingly. But I should have listened to my inner voice then and for a long time afterwards. I never did let Steven in on my darkest desires and hidden truths. For ten years, I kept them safely locked away.

It wasn't that hard to adjust to married life. So many success stories surrounded me. I had a plan. First, the dulling down of my wardrobe. Out went my toys, the leather, and the bold colours; in came the cashmere and the neutrals. Next, I replaced my favourite carnal red nail colour with a taupe one. I drew the line at tossing the sexy expensive underwear; Steven was happy that only he got to enjoy that hidden side of me. Maybe pregnancy softened me. Because in the end I capitulated.

My new persona felt like a watered-down version of my former self. Yet, my family welcomed this new me—this tamed beast.

"Steven has been so good for our Tamsin. It's what she's been missing in her life, what she needs -Stability. We were incredibly relieved that he stepped up to do the right thing."

The twin's birth was a reminder that the wild Tamsin still existed. It felt primal. For those twelve hours of labour, I welcomed the turmoil. It made me feel alive again. With hormones coursing through my body and wracked with pain, I surrendered to the urge to scream through each contraction. Pain relief wasn't an option; I embraced each wave of discomfort. At the end of a protracted and rather complicated delivery, I felt wrung out yet absolved of my sins, a clean slate.

Steven and the children love the new Tamsin. When we entertain at home, I am the quiet one. Steven is our spokesperson, as no one is remotely interested in the bits and bytes of my job, anyway. He holds the floor as he recalls their latest milestones and achievements. He continuously checks in with me but is confident in his role. His self-assurance comes from the mantles he wears; husband, father, and therapist. They suit him. He feels valued. Life is good for him. He has help managing the house. A cleaner, twice a week. I pay for that, the house, and the service. He is popular on the school circuit. I watch him flirt innocently with the mums. They validate his manliness. This life is as good as it will ever be for him. I, on the other hand, can never have it all.

We don't talk about our innermost feelings; we play our respective roles in this life we've carved for ourselves. It's a good life. Anyone looking in will agree. A stable marriage and a loving family are what they see. They don't feel the silence as I do. It consumes me from within. Work is what recharges me and makes coming home possible.

Is this love? We love the children; we make love; we feel loved and cared for. That's enough, isn't it?

For a long time, I carried the trauma of the rape with me as a permanent reminder not to fuck things up. So what if it felt like my spirit was slowly dying? When Julian joined the company as my assistant, I felt the faint stirrings of colour again. I knew that even as a non-executive mother and home maker, I still had my share of responsibilities. Richard, my boss, thought I was juggling too much and insisted I add another head to my team. Many candidates were suitable, but I clicked with Julian straight away. Our connection felt much more than just a professional one. His campness amused me, and his shoot-from-the-hip approach suited my leadership style. We were soon inseparable, both in and out of the office. He proved himself trustworthy and loyal to me on many occasions. He was even stepping in to babysit when we found ourselves at a loss. He liked Steven, and in turn, they all adored him. The twins call him Uncle Jules. Ha, he loves that! But it was *our* connection that mattered most to him. He became my confidant, and I shared details of my sordid past.

"Tamsin, I'm not here to judge you; God knows I have a rather colourful life myself."

While we kept our work relationship strictly professional, after hours, I'd accompany him to gay bars and night clubs. We both worked hard by day, so I felt vindicated on these nights out. I enjoyed the energy, the music, and the dancing. I lived vicariously through his dalliances. He unashamedly left the club with anyone he was attracted to. I envied his freedom. I should have known that I was edging closer to danger. Julian could see that I was trying to be a good wife, and he knew I loved my children. But he also caught glimpses of my flirtatious, wilder side. On these nights out, he watched me play with men. It could go no further than that.

"Maybe you need to do this to be that good person. It satisfies your carnal instincts. For God's sake, don't cross the line."

But I did cross the line.

Mark was a prospective client of ours. He owned a company that was responsible for off-site data storage. He was young and incredibly attractive. Richard and I were wooing him in an attempted takeover bid. He'd visited the offices a few times, and while we were never alone, I always felt his gaze on me.

Later he'd say, "I watched how the skin around your throat would redden. With just a glance, I could make your blood rush to the surface."

Of course, I felt our chemistry. I'd have been a fool not to. That rush, my weakening resolve. I hadn't felt it in ages. It awoke something in me.

"You're the most senior director here, Tamsin. And the most experienced in acquisitions," said Richard. "You take him out to dinner; find out his weaknesses."

Oh shit, here we go again.

The Trellis was where we went. Over two courses and a shared bottle of red wine, I did my job. Over the dessert course and a whiskey, I played my own game in my head. Strength: he smells amazing, something expensive, no doubt. Weakness: he has no idea how attractive he is. Didn't even notice the waitress fawning over him whenever she came to our table.

He held my gaze throughout our meal. His hand would brush mine as he topped up my wine glass. He watched me silently, intently, when I excused myself to visit the powder room. Later he reached over to lift and admire the sailor's knot pendant at my neck, and as his fingers grazed my neck, I was sure he could feel my heart pounding. We didn't want the evening to end, so he suggested we go to a bar for a nightcap. As I stood up he leaned over to help me put on my coat. He slid his arms around my neck, grabbing hold of my hair. Gathering it in one hand, he wound it around slowly and gently while lifting it out. Not breaking contact, he turned me around and stared into the depths of my soul. We didn't make it to the bar.

"How did it go with Mighty Mark last night? You look a bit weary," smirks Julian as we collect our coffees the following day.

"Good, I think he's interesting ... uh interested. Wants to talk to Richard this morning."

"Ha interested in what exactly?" he asks raising his perfectly plucked eyebrow.

"Not now, Julian. It was a business dinner, that's all. Besides, my head is pounding; I didn't sleep well."

"Bet you didn't. As long as *he* didn't make it *his* business to pound you!" Julian says, laughing.

"Don't be crass; now shut up and tell me what I'm doing today."

For now, I'm going to keep what happened my little secret. I felt both ashamed and equally brazen. It took all my junior school drama skills to hide this emotion from Julian. I'm not sure where this tryst will go. I suspect it is a one-off, so in my mind, this little blip never happened. But oh God, it was thrilling and oh so very satisfying. I replay our subsequent evenings repeatedly in my mind, enjoying the warmth and the pulse this creates between my legs.

He checks us into a boutique hotel close by. We collect the key, and chastely we walk to the room. When the door shuts behind us, only then does he reach for me. I brush my lips against his neck while pushing his coat off his broad shoulders. He pulls back slightly, not letting go of me but not wanting to give in to me just yet. I look into his eyes as I slowly start to unbutton his shirt. The muscles of his chest tighten as I run my hand over them. I can feel the proof of his wanting me at the front of his trousers, in every muscle as he attempts to hold himself back. I pull his head down and bring his lips to mine. I run my tongue over them gently before whispering, let's not hold back.

And just like that, we unleash our inner beasts.

Focus Tamsin! Back to reality.

But it wasn't that easy. My thoughts keep straying—another encounter.

I disentangle myself from his embrace and the bedsheets and quietly dress. I look longingly at his sleeping body, wishing I could crawl back into his arms. Once again, stroking the smooth lines of his muscled torso and running my fingers down his happy trail. Feeling his strong arms wrap around me as he joins me. His legs engulfing mine. His hardness to my softness. I have never known such passion and long to experience it again.

I feel wrung out after our sexual encounters. Spent. I love to watch him sleep. Just then, he stirs and opens his eyes. He remains quiet as I calmly gather my things. I see the questions in his penetrating gaze. I blow him a kiss, turn and leave.

Must get home.

I let myself in quietly. Steven knows not to wait up. I go to the cupboard and find the half-empty bottle of wine there. Pouring a large glass, I quickly finish it. I pour another. Compose yourself, Tamsin. I need to wash his smell off me. I methodically start wiping my face, neck, and breasts using wet kitchen towels. Every stroke feels like a further betrayal. I keep wiping and discarding the evidence until I'm satisfied I can go upstairs and climb into bed with my husband again. Steven sleeps on soundly, trustingly.

Mark called me the next day. He'd concluded business with Richard and wanted to celebrate. He didn't appear to mind when I said that Richard would accompany me. Again, we were to go to dinner—he chose the restaurant this time. On the way, I called Steven. I hadn't seen him that day. I'd continued sleeping on even after he'd taken the children to school.

"Don't worry, my love, you must have been knackered," he says. "I understand; this is a big deal for you and Richard. Go ahead. I'll tell the kids' Mum's working hard and will see them at the weekend. Take all the time you need."

I don't deserve him.

I berate myself for all the times I've criticised him—all the horrible thoughts I have in those moments when he clings to me like a baby. I feel disgusted when he sweeps the children's leftovers into his mouth. My unkind remarks about the weight he has put on recently. He jokes about being the human waste disposal. "Makes cleaning up so much easier." None of my barbs find their mark. His default is to shrug and laugh it off.

I don't deserve him.

Richard and I are sitting in a dimly lit Moroccan-style restaurant later. The smells are intoxicating. Mark joins us a few minutes later. "Traffic," he shrugs unapologetically. Our eyes meet. He looks down at the sailor's knot. This gift from my husband. I blush when I think about what he did with it last night. Richard wastes no time and propels us straight into business. I cannot focus, especially when I catch Mark's eye. Maybe it's also how we share platters of delicious food, the smells of the spices wafting around the table. He tears some flatbread and dips it into the hummus before offering it to Richard, who politely declines, and then to me. His fingers deliberately brush my lips, and he laughingly wipes away a crumb that lands on my chin.

Richard is utterly oblivious to the sexual tension at our table. While he peruses the wine list, I feel Mark's hand slide between my legs under the table. At some point slightly flustered, I excuse myself to visit the lady's room. The door opens as I stand in front of the mirror, staring at my reddened cheeks and trying to still my racing heart. It's Mark. He pulls me into a cubicle, locks the door, and kisses me passionately. He exposes my breasts and takes one hardened nipple into his mouth. He spreads my legs with his knee and plunges his hand down the front of my knickers, stroking my slick core. As I climax, he covers my mouth with his own and swallows my moans. I cling to him as wave after wave of unadulterated pleasure washes over me. Then, forsaking his own, he smiles at me, takes a deep breath, adjusts his erection, and just as discretely, he leaves. It takes a while for my rush to subside.

We are back at the table, making sure to have arrived separately. Without missing a beat, Richard continues with business, stopping briefly to ask, "Are you all right, Tamsin? You must be coming down with something. You look a bit flushed."

An ecstasy of orgasms later and with all our project deadlines put to bed, I finally agreed to meet Julian at his flat for a quick catchup. As I ride the lift to the top floor, I study my face in the mirror. Work stress has taken its toll, my eyes feel dry, but I still look and feel incredible. I was meeting Mark straight after, so I had dressed for that date. Julian will never guess that I am Mistress Tamsin beneath this demure cashmere dress. My shoulder bag carries everything I need for the occasion.

"Glass of wine?" Asks Julian as I make myself comfortable on his designer sofa. "So babe, about that mindfuck comment you dropped the other day. Are you ready to spill the beans?"

Taking a big gulp, liquid courage, and all that, I tell Julian about Mark and me, that we're having an affair. I confide to him about our instant attraction. "I'm in trouble, Jules," I tell him everything.

"You don't have to explain to me, hun. I was there! He looked at you like a dog looks at a bitch on heat. Oh, to be on the receiving end of those dark smouldering eyes."

"Should I be concerned that he's so young? And that he's not married?"

"Hell no, you're the only unfaithful one. Besides, when has that ever stopped you?"

Taking a big sip of wine, I go quiet.

"What's going on? What's bugging you?"

It's probably nothing, but Mark had asked me why I removed my wedding band when we were together. I wasn't even aware that I was doing this. Now I wonder what that means for him or, more importantly, for Steven.

"Hun, I'm no therapist, but it appears you have feelings for both. Removing your band is your subconscious mind, compartmentalising each relationship. So now all you have to work out is which one matters more. But enough of that, tell me about the sex."

Mark makes me feel like the old Tamsin. I feel alive when I'm with him. I've even started wearing my favourite red nail varnish again. The sex is incredible. "He's up for the BDSM stuff. He's happy to indulge my darkest fantasies. I never have to fake orgasms with him."

"Fake orgasms! That is just scandalous! Why the hell would you need to do that? I thought Steven was a generous lover."

He is, well, he was. We haven't slept together in a while now, actually, for as long as I've been seeing Mark. "By the way, I only faked it when I was tired."

"So why leave? Steven is your comfort blanket. He'll always be there, faithful to a fault, and he adores you. Why not have the best of both? Couples are considering thruples these days. It's a thing."

"It's not *my* thing; besides, it's unfair to Steven." We've given each other a decade. He deserves to be considered and let down gently. I'm unsure how to begin our uncoupling or what I'd even say to him. "I worry that I'm going to lose my best friend."

"I thought I was your best friend," says Julian petulantly. "But I do know what you mean. Much like your husband, I am now competing with Mighty Mark for your precious time and attention. But not your body!"

"Fuck off, Julian!" I have always been logical. A thrill seeker certainly. My success is driven by these traits. And I have never let my emotions get the better of me. So this state of inner turmoil is troubling. "My heart and mind are in constant battle, and my body seems to have a will of its own."

"That body is getting laid, good and proper!"

I haven't had a proper period in months. Patchy at best. At first, I thought I was pregnant, but subsequent tests have revealed otherwise. As a result of work stress and a busy mind, I'm not sleeping well. And I'm constantly flushing, even when Mark's not around.

"Flushes, anxiety, insomnia, you sound like my mother!"

I have scheduled another doctor's appointment next week. So I'll know more then.

"What a relief you're not pregnant. Babies clash with project deadlines."

So what is going on with me? I feel like I'm unravelling.

He takes his phone out and starts scrolling. "Brace yourself, hun; you're not going to like this. The almighty Google says, based on your age and your symptoms, you're in premature menopause," says Julian, revealing the contents of his search.

Oh shit! But I'm only thirty-nine. What does that even mean?

| 3 |

Let's talk about your privates.

Welcome back.

Thank you for tuning in again, ladies. Without further ado...*let's talk about your privates.*

We know that sex is important. The question is: Do you still want it? Can you still have it? Can you get there?

What are the obstacles to having a good sex life in the middle years and beyond? Health issues? Hormonal issues? Partner issues?

With me today is our favourite TV gynaecologist, Barry Glover, here to answer your more physiological submissions, while Mistress Precious Payne, founder and owner of the Pleasure Palace, is our expert in all things sexual.

Let's go to our first submission. This one goes to the panel.

My libido is waning. Finding it harder to reach climax. I'm no longer in sync with my partner. Is this it? Is it goodbye sex life?

Barry: Libido can be affected by smoking, alcohol, gynaecological surgeries, and medications such as anti-depressants.

Jane: So how is that relevant for a menopausal woman?

Barry: Well, it's all to do with the exciter hormone, oestrogen, and it's declining levels. That doesn't mean to say that your libido is lost and that climax is impossible. The mechanisms are still there; it's how you maintain their working order.

Jane: Barry, are you talking about hormonal creams, rings, patches, and pessaries?

Barry: Yes, these have proven successful in many patients; however, libido is an emotional response. Perhaps Precious wants to weigh in on that.

Precious: I agree. Sexual desire has many contributing factors. Besides health and medication, emotional responses are often linked to relationship strain, stress, and anxiety.

Jane: Statistics show that the highest divorce rate belongs to the middle years. As a divorcee, I felt my relationship had reached its sell-by date. In more ways than one.

Precious: Without relationship crimes, you can reverse boredom with new forms of play, different toys – different rules. Couples' landscapes change.

Jane: Do you feel that the older generation knows what they want? Are they more self-assured?

Precious: Absolutely. My clients have already worked out what they like, and they own it.

Jane: You've previously mentioned using toys and role-play to spice things up in the bedroom. Is this the age of creativity?

Precious: Without the fear of pregnancy, many women do feel liberated. Many couples have introduced a third party into the bedroom and often joke they're going to bed with Wilbur, Moby (Dick), or Roger. The dildo squad.

Barry: Without being the voice of gloom and doom, along with liberation, midlife patients throw caution to the wind and are shocked when they discover how many sexually transmitted diseases are doing the rounds.

Jane: In these new relationships, why aren't we insisting on condoms?

Barry: Well, as the token middle-aged man here, I can confirm that condoms mean safe sex, yet there is a fear of deflation and loss of sensation, all of which contribute to performance anxiety.

Precious: This is still the age of desire, arousal, and climax, just not in double-quick time. It's more about lingering, indulging, and luxuriating in all-consuming erotic conversations.

Jane: You make that sound incredibly sensual and appetising. Are we talking massage, candles, and aromatherapy or lip licking, chocolate dripping and so on?

Precious: Ha-ha, all of the above.

Jane: Now let's step it up a gear. This question from another listener,

"I enjoy rough sex; what advice would you give me as I start my menopausal journey?"

Precious: It depends on how you define rough sex. It can be anything from tickling, playful spanking, and hair pulling to slapping, whipping, and choking. None of these especially relate to the sexual organs. It's a power play build-up. The arousal triggers the power dynamic, or vice versa. Pain is relative, and whether you are inflicting or receiving it, both parties must agree on the rules.

Jane: Painful intercourse is a common complaint, though. Are we talking more than lubrication here, or is this the start of vaginal atrophy?

Barry: Both are correct. One of the more common conditions in peri-and-postmenopausal women is pelvic floor hypertonus; quite simply, the vagina says "NO!" It's to do with the involuntary tightening of the muscles around the vagina in response to pain triggered by entry. It's one part of the genitourinary syndrome of menopause.

Jane: Is that what's known as GSM Barry? If so, that is a relatively recent term.

Barry: Yes, that's right. It's an umbrella term for symptoms in the genitals and lower urinary tract caused by reduced oestrogen levels. Genital atrophy encompasses thinning, drying, and irritation, causing painful sex and urinary tract infections.

Jane: So why the constant infections?

Barry – Because lower oestrogen levels have a knock-on effect of decreasing glycogen levels from the vaginal epithelium, the pH levels are out of whack, causing lactobacillus levels to proliferate. As many as forty per cent of menopausal women will have recurrent UTIs. As you age, the risk of UTIs increases, and with atrophy and reduced sensation, the symptoms may present differently. Urine testing kits are readily available and will confirm any UTIs rather than anything more sinister.

Precious: Yes Barry. Sex at all ages will require a level of care and careful management. Clean the toys and pee after sex to flush out that area. Also, watch what you put in your bath water.

Jane: Talking about painful sex and UTIs. Getting fruity after a chilli festival is a no-no. Trust me. It will feel like the grim reaper has arrived. If you didn't know before, you'd soon realise that certain regions are now more sensitive.

Precious: Ouch, that has me crossing my legs. I can only imagine the screams being louder than the ambulance's sirens.

Jane: And speaking of crossing one's legs, over to you, Barry.

Barry: That's right, Jane. Urinary incontinence is another component of GSM.

Jane: This brings us to our final question.

"I suffer from incontinence. It's so embarrassing. Will it get worse?"

Barry: There are two types of incontinence: *Stress* and *Urge*. The stress type is caused by laughing, coughing, sneezing, lifting heavy objects, and so forth.

Jane: Excuse me, Barry, I've got to cut in here because we can all relate to this. Ladies, I'm sure you've looked at the trampoline longingly but know you can't go there. Think of ever spreading dark grey patches on light grey leggings with every bounce. It's not a pretty sight.

Precious: Let's not forget that any loss of control can result in a spurt, plus an overwhelming need to pee immediately. A pleasant or unpleasant experience, depending on the context.

Barry: Ah, yes, I see. Well, that overwhelming need is urge incontinence—the urgency of this need; and the fear of losing control.

Jane: I'm not alone in thinking we've all been there too. It's that dash to a busy public loo. You're waiting, hopping from side to side, hands crossed in the fig leaf position. *Get ready.* You start unbuckling the belt, quickly releasing the top button. Suddenly the door opens, and you're off. Bouldering in, banging the door shut. *Get set.* Handbag. Floor? Too disgusting. No, Hook. Drop the pants. *And go.* Pivot, aim and fire. And the added insult of the tell-tale patches which show up the betrayal of your pelvic muscles.

Precious: What's the alternative? Because incontinence pull-ups with reinforcements are not sexy at all. Plus, they're costly.

Barry: Yes, incontinence is a taboo topic, and advertisers will have you believe it is inevitable for middle-aged women. *It is not!* There are many things you can do: lifestyle changes such as limiting caffeine and alcohol intake, pelvic floor exercises with Kegel balls, bladder training, and of course, weight management. In more severe cases, surgical intervention and medication are also options.

Jane: Bottom line, don't be a victim, do something about it.

Barry: Correct.

Precious: I couldn't agree more. Incontinence needn't be inevitable. That is very reassuring.

Jane: Enough about our privates; let's talk sexual intimacy. Precious, as an expert in all things sexual, what are your top tips for lust and love in our middle years?

Precious: It's less about 'push here, stroke there, tweak this, slap that.' Arousal may be a series of rolling hills rather than building up to a dramatic peak. Instead, it's about a deeper connection with your partner, with mutual awareness being the end goal. Think tantric sex, a slow, meditative approach to sex with the end goal not necessarily being orgasm but enjoying the journey and all the sensations of the whole body along the way.

Jane: Maybe not the all-day version. Ouchy. A study of five hundred heterosexual couples measuring the time of sex from penetration to ejaculation lasts, on average, 5.4 minutes. So how much time are we talking about for your exploratory meditation session?

Precious: Well, further studies confirm what I've always known; it takes a woman, on average, 12 to just over 14 minutes to reach orgasm. So, this suggests that if we take a longer, more sensual route, the orgasm becomes a consequence rather than the focus and puts the female at centre stage.

Jane: If this is a different approach, where do we start?

Precious: Well, to start, couples need to find a comfortable space and look for novelty, not predictable patterns. Comfort is vital; however, consider taking it out of the bedroom. Create your safe space together. Allow her to determine her level of exposure.

Jane: Are there any body positions that you'd recommend?

Precious: We're not talking about the Kama Sutra; instead, any position that allows her pleasure points to be the focus.

Jane: So clitoral stimulation, then?

Precious: Mostly yes. With its eight thousand nerve endings, the clitoris is the female powerhouse of pleasure. For this exercise, though, all the focus should be on the north-eastern region of the bulb. Using one hand to apply pressure onto the lower groin while continuing to massage with the other, the other partner can elevate the level of sensation. All the while remaining fully aware of the feedback, she communicates with her hand on their leg. It is a journey of intimacy for the couple. How long this continues is entirely the woman's decision.

Jane: So an unfinished story is possible. Perhaps to be continued at another time?

Precious: Indeed. Pleasure will follow when women take centre stage and are no longer just the supporting role.

Jane: You're awfully quiet, Barry. Anything to add?

Barry: What an interesting discussion this has been. Mmm, so foreplay needs to be longer?

Precious: Afraid so, Barry, and let's not forget after-play too.

Jane: Absolutely; the afterglow lasts much longer if the affection continues. So, choose your loo moment wisely.

Well, listeners, I think you'll agree that this has been a rather titillating discussion and an excellent way to end this **talk about your privates.** Thank you to our lovely guests for their knowledge and insight.

Remember to change the pace; it's not a race!

Tune into our next podcast, where we examine the voices in your head.

Until then,

Goodbye.

| 4 |

Fiona's story

"Ok ladies, my next one, I've decided, is going on my inner right wrist, and it's going to be a multi-coloured, …wait for it…PARA-CHUTE".

I announced to my two besties, my 'Charlie's Angels.'

Whenever I call them that, they respond together and shout, "Who the hell is Charlie?" it's been a running laugh since my hen night years ago.

"Let's drink to that," said Kim. "At last, it's taken you ages to make your mind up, Fi."

"Another bottle of bubbles please."

"I know," I said, "but it's painful, Kim. I need to get it right. It's going to be symbolic of a new chapter in my life." I didn't want another bloody flower. If anyone had suggested a poppy, I would have screamed.

My new tattoo had to compliment my other one on the inner side of my left wrist, my marriage hand. It was a daisy, and Lee and I had chosen it together. Or rather, he chose the flower.

"If we have matching daisies inside our wrists on our marriage hands, at the hospice, they will know that you belong to me, and I belong to you." He said, "think about it, Fi, we can wave each other off, Daisy-to-Daisy." I started to tear up as I didn't find it funny, but neither did he really.

"And if they don't bury me properly, Fi, and you recognise my hand, you can complain that your husband is literally pushing up daisies."

It was our private joke and our way of coping with his diagnosis that his cancer had come back, and it was terminal.

It was my first tattoo. I hated most of Lee's, especially the Arsenal one. The gun or cannon was lopsided and showed no skill. "Just like your tattoo, mate, no skill," his best friend Paul, also known as 'One-Nerve,' teased when their club played badly. One-Nerve was a good friend and solid most of the time, but he had a trip switch. He would go quiet, and anyone else on-site knew to steer clear. And when he said, "I've got just one nerve, mate, and you're standing on it," you knew that if the guy it was aimed at didn't back off, a punch would follow. When Lee's diagnosis came, Paul disappeared behind our house and sobbed.

I was right, having it done *was* bloody painful. It felt like a sort of test, a kind of ceremony. I hoped that the outcome, the daisy, would be pretty and clean looking, not grubby. It was. Lee wanted the same design but not filled, just a black–ink sketch. He thought it was more manly looking that way.

I said thank God he hadn't wanted a barcode tattooed on his left big toe so the mortuary could scan him and tick 'dispatched.' We had a lot of dark- humour days. It was everyone's way of coping.

I was relieved that my tattoo was exactly what I wanted. It was pretty and clean-looking, and I wore it with pride. It would be my lasting tribute to Lee and a lasting memory for me. But, unfortunately, we had to get his done quickly as his treatment was about to begin.

As he went through agony, having my first tattoo was my way of sharing his pain. It felt right. Most of my friends had them anyway, so I was just joining the club. It was going to be my badge of honour.

He cried too when we were both having them done. We both realised that this would be the beginning of the end.

How weak he looked. It was hard to believe that this man of mine, who was so strong, so loud, and such a clown, had been reduced to this.

Mind you, I paid the price too. As he got thinner, I got fatter, and being short and round was no longer 'cute.' I wasn't his pocket rocket anymore. But he still loved me, he had to; I was his carer. No, that's not fair. We were each other's love, and although he wasn't a saint, I knew he loved me. I was his, quiet-before-a-glass gal, then three drinks in, I became his 'Fearless-Fi.'

I met Lee at a festival. I was twenty-two, working in events, and he was thirty-eight and the sparky on-site, doing the rigging. He looked me up and down, winked, smiled, and said, "Alright?" I thought he was so sexy but also such a lad. A really Cheeky Chappie, with the gift of the gab. He found it easy to flirt whilst I felt just shy. He said, "Hi there, is that you?" I said, "What do you mean?" And he said, "The person who smells nice?" "Maybe", I replied, and he said back, "So she smells nice *and* is cute." I blushed. I felt cute when he said it. So our love story began. I had been on the pill for a few years and had a couple of relationships, a few holiday romances and one major heartbreak. But Lee got me in a way that made me super confident when I was with him and paranoid when I was without him.

He was divorced and a bit bitter when we met. His ex had gone off with their two sons to America, so he never saw them.

My girlfriends thought he was gorgeous but dangerous too. They also thought he was totally into me. I was cautious when we first started going out. I was a good girl from a close family. I loved my mum and dad, and my older sister was my best friend. She warned, "Go carefully with him. I think he's a bit of a tart," so I did. I didn't want his friends to think that I was easy. I made him wait. When we eventually had sex, it was amazing. I knew I was right; he knew what he was doing. He was a cheeky cock and always fun. But then I kept getting thrush, so he offered to take himself off to the Gum clinic to get checked out. He got the all-clear, and I said that was sweet of him and showed that he cared. Then he said, "Yes, I do, I love you, and I thought it wouldn't be fair on you if I passed any-thing on." I asked how many women he had shagged, and he told me straight, "Since I was fifteen? Before you, about two hundred." I said that was disgusting, but thought, not surprised, women seemed to turn to jelly around him.

We started living with each other, and he was house-trained. He had his rough work clothes but then changed into a peacock with his fancy shirts at the weekend. Our gang grew, and his lads teamed up with my girlfriends. It was a life full of laughter and occasional tears.

When I turned twenty-eight, I was beginning to fret that he was just using me. My dad wanted him to make an honest woman of me. I said that I thought it was old-fashioned, but my girlfriends got engaged and married one by one, and I felt left out waiting for a proposal.

One hen night in Amsterdam, I met a younger version of Lee, and at a nightclub, we got off with each other. I didn't feel guilty; in fact, it was my right. There were more fish in the sea and all that. If Lee couldn't commit, he would miss out. But the guy seemed too keen and serious, so I blew him off. When I got home, Lee had missed me. His lads came around, and their playful teasing and sense of humour seduced me again. "No, that's Stabbing-Nigel." "Why is he called Stabbing-Nigel?" I asked, fearful of another violent character. "Darlin, we call him stabbing because his surname is Payne – the stabbing pain, boring. Always wittering on about health and safety all the time. So we send him off to collect the ladder with wheels." They roared with laughter. I thought, *You sod, you win me over every time.*

We still don't know whether Nigel ever understood the lads' nicknames of the two identical twins. One being frigid and the other being easy, as 'Stop' and 'Go.'

Eventually, all our friends partnered up and got married. First, Leanne and Nigel. Next, Kim and One-Nerve. Finally, at this last wedding, Lee proposed. I was already tearful, having watched Kim and One-Nerve get hitched. One-Nerve said in his speech that he knew straight away that Kim was the perfect match for him when they met in the pub. He admired the rabbit brooch on her jumper and said, "I bet I could make that bunny hop," as he put his hand under her left boob, she immediately said, "I bet I could make you hop higher" and went to knee him in his groin.

That day we'd stayed at the hotel and were both hung over. Lee ordered room service. I'd lost my appetite, but Lee insisted that we have breakfast and that I had to lift the silver platter. And there it was, a ring made out of electric cable with a note.

Fi, we're electric together, I may be the sparky, but you are my spark. Marry me, my little pocket rocket?

(Oh yeah, and choose your own ring – I'll cock it up)

I'd never been happier. I couldn't stop crying, and we couldn't stop hugging each other.

We went through the usual hen and stag nights and had a lovely wedding by the sea. On my honeymoon, I felt sick and had a miscarriage. That was surprising, as we hadn't even talked about trying for children. Two more gut punches followed: one, Lee was more relieved than sorry about the miscarriage; two, the paragliding that we had booked, had to be cancelled. So, a double loss and a bit of a shitty ending to the honeymoon. Never mind, we had a nice tan to prove to our friends that we had a wonderful time.

The loss of a potential baby made my body clock go into turbo drive. If I hadn't wanted one before, I wanted a baby now. Lee was less keen. He said that he'd be too old, an ancient dad. He wouldn't feel happy on a pitch teaching a son football at his age. His older boys were in their late twenties by now and soon would be fathers themselves. He'd probably be a granddad before he would be a father again. It was all too weird. I cried a river, and every time one of my girlfriends had a baby, Lee and I had a row. In the end, he gave in, and after a year of trying, I fell pregnant.

I had an easy pregnancy, and after the first twelve weeks of feeling awful, I enjoyed it. Lee kept telling me that he thought I looked gorgeous. We had a very sexy time until the last month.

The birth was bloody horrendous—the worse 36 hours of my life. I was exhausted, and the tearing of my undercarriage didn't bare thinking about. All I can say is that I felt undone and thought I'd never be the same again.

Baby Molly was beautiful, but I was frightened of everything and out of control. Mum and my sister were brilliant, but I just couldn't get a grip. Molly was easy as babies go, so I felt ungrateful. Lee stayed away a lot of the time as he said I was "scary" during this time. My friends came around, and we had baby sessions together, but it felt weird and surreal. I was going mad. My mum moved in as I wasn't sleeping, I became obsessed about cleaning the house, but I looked like shit. I wouldn't let Lee anywhere near Molly. He could do nothing right. I can't even remember this period. It was one big blur. I just remember thinking that it was never going to end. It was really gloomy, and I would never be my old self and happy ever again.

Lee was very irritated and intolerant most of the time. He muttered that he'd wished we had never had Molly; we were happy before she came along. I felt even more guilty and thought, *be careful what you wish for.* Thankfully, when Molly turned one, my depression lifted, and Lee fell in love with his daughter. Her chuckles had him wrapped around all of her little fingers. His little princess could do no wrong. We agreed to stop at one, and I was never going to go through that nightmare again. It was really frightening, and it didn't do our marriage any good at all.

I gave up work to be a stay-at-home mum, and his business with One-Nerve Paul was doing well. When we had the money, we would spend it. Molly was getting quite spoiled. Our group would have Spanish holidays together. Life was good.

I started looking after myself again, having my hair and nails done, all-over spray tan (Lee hated the smell). Then, going out shopping with the girls and after a couple of years, when our kids were all through the toddler years, and if my mum could do the babysitting (Lee's mum and dad weren't interested, they felt too old), the 'Charlie's Angels' started to have girlie weekends away again. It was our time, the spa weekends.

The boys also went on their lads' away weekends, usually involving football matches and far too many beers. All of us had drunken antics but harmless. There were a few casualties in our group. Kim and One-Nerve went through a difficult patch, but I hoped Lee and I had served our time and earned our stripes in our marriage with the post-natal. But then I had to see the doctor about a gynae problem, I was spotting in between periods and after sex, and I had a funny pain in my tummy. I was worried but devastated when the doctor said I had an STD. I'd only been with Lee since I turned twenty-two, and all the tests when I was pregnant with Molly, were clear.

Lee was cheating, and I wanted to know who with. I told him what the doctor said, and he put his head in his hands and said, "Sorry, babe, I don't even remember her name; I was wasted." I shouted, "I'm grateful that it was just chlamydia. It could have been much worse: herpes, Aids, whatever. Your fucking ego could have killed me!" I was furious, and he knew it. My sister was furious too, and we agreed Mum and Dad mustn't find out. It took a while. Lee had to wear the shame for six weeks. He cried buckets and promised never to risk losing Molly and me ever again. So I eventually forgave him. I was actually relieved that it was just a one-night stand as a couple of our pack who had affairs were really suffering when their marriages broke.

Us girls knew that the boys were no angels, but we just hoped that they all loved us too much to do anything stupid. One by one, the cracks in all our marriages began to show. Most of us patched things up and kept going. The pack was stronger than the couples, and we kept each other in check.

As the Charlie's Angels got older, we became louder and more flirtatious. We all thought our men were great and also pathetic. It was like having another child. But we were all fond of each other and loyal.

I felt free when I got my coil (my doctor told me I'd been on the pill for too many years). Lee said he could feel the threads but was just showing off. A couple of months went by, and I started to smell like a fish shop down there. It was embarrassing. I felt worried and thought Lee had been cheating again. It turned out that the coil just hadn't suited me. The doctor said that it had interrupted my ph balance and BV *(BTM: Bacterial Vaginosis)* was the reason for the smell. Course after course of antibiotics happened. I couldn't wait for menopause, and then I could give up any form of contraception and go 'Au Naturelle.' Or maybe Lee could have the snip. I mentioned it to Lee, and he went quiet. I said it was easier for him to have the snip than for me to be sterilised.

I asked if he was frightened of not being able to get a stiffy again. Or did he think it would make him any less of a man. He admitted that he'd already had it done years ago. It turned out that he had done it behind my back when I was suffering from the post-natal. I was livid. He said that he did it for me, but I doubted that. He had done it for himself and hadn't run it by me. How dare he! What if I had wanted another baby? I didn't, but that wasn't the point. He had watched me continue to take the pill and then get a coil fitted and not said a word, bloody coward. He'd been sneaky, and I wondered what else he had done behind my back without my say-so. He broke my trust again, and I was never going to let him forget it.

It had an impact on me and Kim's relationship too; she must have known as One-Nerve was Lee's best friend. She said that she had no idea, and she was sure that Paul didn't know anything about it either. So Lee was called Sneak for a while. In a way, he'd betrayed us all.

Then Leanne found a lump in her breast. The Charlie's Angels took the news as a team and gathered around. It was a terrible two years for everyone. The boys were tamed too, and we had many discussions about how when one in our pack is hurting, it hurts everyone. Leanne had to lose the actual breast and go through the hell of the chemo. It shocked us all, and each couple was so grateful that it wasn't any one of us, but also, we felt the guilt of why not us? Leanne's breast augmentation was great; we all joked about it being the best boob job ever. We made cherry Bakewell cupcakes with a cherry on top to celebrate when she got the 'all clear.' We also learned how to wear a wig, tie scarves around our heads, draw natural eyebrows (a mixture of brown and grey pencils), and create natural-looking eyelashes; cheap falsies cut in half and only applied to each eye's middle and outer half. Stuff we hoped we didn't need to know, but we did it anyway. Supporting each other as if we were all going through it ourselves. Our pack always tried to find the humour in everything, but this time it was hard. We dug deep as if our own lives depended on it.

When Leanne was cancer free, the Charlie's Angels booked a celebration. Another spa weekend, this time on the Isle of Wight, and it was just what the doctor ordered. We did gentle walks, heart-to-heart chats, swimming, and three treatments each. We went to a nice restaurant, just a stone's throw from the hotel, and got plastered. Leanne wanted an early night, so we walked her back. Kim and I went straight back to the bar. We both got chatted up by two middle-aged lads who had been in a squash tournament. It was so good feeling wanted again. The four of us then went on to a nightclub and boogied the night away. Kim threw up after her fourth cocktail, so my guy and I took her back to the hotel. His mate bailed. "I don't do vomit." Once Kim was through the door of our bedroom, my guy pounced. It was strange but nice to be kissed and fumbled by a stranger. I felt young again. He grabbed my hand and led me to his room at the end of the corridor.

It was fast and clumsy. His cock wasn't as good as Lee's, but the act felt familiar. I felt like I'd been in a movie, and it wasn't happening to me. His wedding ring made me think, *Poor cow, I wonder if his wife knows what he gets up to.* But I had no guilt. As I stumbled along the corridor back to our girls' room, I hoped that I'd got away with it. That is when the guilt caught up with me: the fear of being found out. Luckily, the other two were snoring as I let myself in with the room key card. I tip-toed to the bathroom, sat on the loo, and thought I must get myself checked out when we all got home. I also needed the morning-after-pill because I couldn't remember if he used something. I had wanted to shower but still felt a bit sick. So I had a quick flannel wash and hoped the girls wouldn't smell him on me. We all joke about cum-n-bare smell.

I went out in the morning to get some ST's *(BTM: Sanitary Towels)* but was happy that the chemist didn't ask too many questions when I asked for the 'magic pill'. What an idiot I had been. Back home, my doctor just got on with the swabs; we'd been here before. All clear. No nasties. Life got back to normal.

When our Molly turned sixteen, she went to a music festival and celebrated her great GCSE results. She was going to go places as she had done much better than her mum and dad. We were so proud. Her antics made all of us feel old. We could barely remember Live Aid. Me and the Charlie's Angels wanted to go to our own festival now. The boys were not interested, but us girls thought we would give it a go, so we booked into a local B&B. Very civilized. I certainly didn't like the sound of the muddy tents, drugs and stepping in another camper's poo as you stepped out of your tent. Which is how Molly described the festival she went to. It sounded disgusting. We weren't going to try any drugs, just stuck to our usual wine, Prosecco, and if we were really going to push the boat out, maybe a few cocktails. Kim and I don't even remember having the blue crystal nose piercings, but we thought they were cool.

When we got home, the boys and our kids thought our nose studs were 'sad' because they practically shouted mid-life crisis. Kim and I felt judged. But sod it, we were planning to grow old, disgracefully.

I wasn't going to admit but the festival made me feel my age. Being so short, the last festival I went to (nothing like the one's today, much smaller and tamer by comparison), I was lifted up and parked on a stranger's shoulders to see the acts on stage. But at this festival, Kim and I thought we were more like Weeble's who wobble but don't fall down. It would take two guys to get us up on their shoulders. Anyway, we had no offers. Gone were those days. We vowed to go back to our slimming clubs and get our act together again.

Molly did well in her A-levels and was the first in our family to go to university. It cost a bloody fortune to get the stuff for her student flat. But it was horrible coming home to a house without her. Luckily, she felt homesick and wanted to come home often in the first year. Lee was more worried about his little girl than I was. Molly had an old head on young shoulders. When she went interrailing around Europe, we knew she had caught the wanderlust bug and hoped she wouldn't want to work abroad after graduating.

My fiftieth birthday came and went. The Charlie's Angels had all gone to our slimming clubs so we felt on top form. Then my joker of a husband decided to lark about posing like Usain Bolt on top of a ladder. His fall pulled umpteen ligaments, and, quick as a flash, we lost our income. We were broke. I was livid again. Thank goodness for One-Nerve helping us out until Lee could get back on his feet. Happy special birthday to me! I don't think so.

In Molly's second year, Lee and I snatched a romantic weekend away in our caravan in Norfolk. When we got home, we found a message on our answering machine. It was the doctor's surgery; something had turned up in Lee's blood tests when he had gone for his follow-up.

We were to phone the surgery immediately. The GP said she was sending an ambulance urgently to take us to hospital. The drama frightened both of us. Test after test in the hospital confirmed that Lee had leukaemia. We stared in disbelief at each other. Then we went silent, asked the doctor many questions, and asked them all again. We were absolutely exhausted. The chemotherapy was to begin immediately as this type, usually found more in children, was extremely aggressive. Lee managed to say, "Mostly found in children? – that'll be the right one for me then." but it wasn't funny, and the doctors had heard all the weak gags before.

When we got home, we hugged and cried. We vowed to throw everything at it, and we'd be damned if cancer was to get in the way; we'd fight it to the bitter end. Molly came home and became hysterical. It was a long and hard weekend. We were all losing the plot. Just as we'd pull ourselves together, we'd all collapse into a heap of tears again. One-Nerve and Kim came over, but they couldn't settle or even look Lee in the eye. Lee noticed that One-Nerve was uncomfortable. I reassured him that Paul would come around. He was just in shock and frightened too. They were best friends, close like brothers. The whole gang got together, but the jokes, for a while, disappeared.

We both immediately tried to stop smoking. It was hard. Especially going to the hospital where groups of patients in wheelchairs were always in front of the doors getting their fix. Getting passed them without breathing in their smoke was torture, but we were determined to kick the habit.

It was good that Molly was at university when the chemo started; she was a one-less person to worry about. It was brutal. Lee had already rung around the gang saying his sweet nothings and farewells in case he didn't make it. The scary part was when nine other medics stood around his bed, some with paddles waiting to resuscitate him if the infusion stopped his heart.

"More volts, please Boris," he said with more courage than his face showed. He was terrified. The young doctors didn't know who Boris Karlov's Frankenstein was; they didn't get the joke. All they managed were polite smiles, but Lee felt he was grabbing at part of his old self.

A few weeks later, he turned yellow with Jaundice, and the gang asked, "How's Bart Simpson today, Fi?" I replied, "Never mind your Bart, it's Homer I'm pushing around in a wheelchair. He may be weak, but he weighs a ton. Feel free to help, lads."

When Lee finished his Chemotherapy and Radiotherapy, our gang clubbed together and fitted a wet room with a chair. Lee was overcome with emotion and couldn't think of anything to say except that I would benefit, too, as his old lady was having more hot flushes than he was. I laughed, but I'm not sure that I noticed how often I was in flames. I was too focused on his treatment. It felt right that it was all about him.

However, I did notice that my language was getting worse. I knew I was stressed. Who wouldn't be? When I went to get a verruca in my foot cut out, I said no to the anaesthetic. After all, my Lee was being brave, so I would be brave too. The nurse started to cut away, and I immediately shouted, "Jesus! What are you doing? Digging it out with a fucking spoon?" She looked shocked, "Sorry," I said. After that, we agreed this was not the time to be brave. Too much going on. And then I told her about my recent panic attack. She suggested I talk to my GP, and so that's when I started on the 'happy pills.'

And still, I refused help. I would look after my husband and protect his dignity. We were a team. I did keep wishing for an electric wheelchair, but they were heavy; too heavy for a 5ft girl to get in and out of the car.

Lee lost all his hair but friends, who had been through chemo, told him that it would grow back thicker, or maybe curly. The jokes were thick too, and maybe too many of them from his mates. "Tried that shampoo? 'Wash and it's gone,' or the Anti-dandruff version, 'Go polish your head.'" One-Nerve knew how sick Lee felt. We both did our best to keep things positive, but it was hard. I was knackered and felt guilty that I was complaining when I wasn't the one going through the hell of the treatments. The cures seemed worse than the illness. It was tough, but Lee didn't feel tough himself. One day he said, "Fi, I feel broken, I'm done."

I said, "You're so close, baby, one more treatment to get to the other side."

I went for a walk to get a cup of tea but slid down the wall in the corridor. I couldn't stop the tears, they had got a hold, and I was sobbing. It was so embarrassing. I'd lost control. An old lady, another visitor, just stooped and patted my back. Her act of kindness made me howl. "Let it all out, sweetheart; it'll pass," and she walked on. I nodded my head but didn't look up. I never did get her name or thank her; maybe she was an angel with hidden wings.

We both held hands in the hospital and didn't speak for ages.

"How is my little pocket rocket? What will you do, Fi, if I make it but never feel the urge to, you know, again? I'll be useless."

"One thing at a time, Mr Sexy." It may be the time for the longest foreplay. "Maybe I could get a vibrator?" I said. "Not funny!" he said.

"Kim swears by hers if she can't swear at One-Nerve".

"Really?" he looked surprised and then smiled awkwardly.

Maybe that had been too much personal information on his mate.

So I lightened the moment by saying, "Yes, it's like that joke, 'A girl doesn't need the whole pig if all she wants is a sausage from time to time.'"

"Your girls' humour is worse than us boys."

Lee's libido was dead, but thankfully, he was not. The recovery from the treatments was slow, really slow. Thank God for his mates. One-Nerve Paul did all the heavy lifting while Lee slowly got back to work. He didn't want to retire. It was good for him to feel normal again: keeping busy and telling tales from each job. He felt guilty about sharing equal money with Paul when he didn't feel like he had been pulling his weight. Paul didn't mind. He was just pleased to get his mate back. In Lee's absence, Stabbing-Nigel had driven him mad.

Lee's check-ups were going well. His hair did grow back, which was funny as mine was beginning to thin. He was still tired and couldn't concentrate for long periods.

Life was back to normal-ish. Molly got a job in hospitality in France, working in a really lovely chateau Hotel. She met and married a French man, Phillipe, the hotel's chef, and Lee and the boys went on a booze cruise to get wine for her wedding. Talk about 'taking coals back to Newcastle.'

The Charlie's Angels and I went back to our slimming clubs. Three of us had put on so much weight; Leanne stayed skinny. Good job that she was so nice; otherwise, we would have hated her, and she'd been through the hell of cancer. Anyway, we just loved her.

My hot flushes were as bad as ever, but I'd rather have those than Kim's headaches and mood swings. One-Nerve had his work cut out at home, for sure. I had my teeth whitened and couldn't stop smiling to show them off. Molly came home for a visit and kept wearing her sunglasses to make the point that my teeth were now too white. So I kept eating chocolate in front of her "just to muddy them up for you, Madam, you understand?" I said.

Time ticked by, and Lee retired officially but did odd jobs for cash. Then we had a double celebration; Lee got the 'all clear,' and our Molly was pregnant. A beautiful baby boy, Marcel, arrived to turn our world upside down. Molly stayed in France, so we nipped over for a visit. Lee was more besotted than the mother. When we got back, he would bore anyone who listened about Marcel's antics. I felt older than my years, knowing I had a grandson. Lee always forgot that I was years younger than him and didn't want to slow down. The Charlie's Angels still wanted to kick up their heels and party. Lee found our loud gatherings irritating. I didn't know whether it was the leftover from his cancer treatment or the fact that I was married to an older man. He'd always been a larger-than-life character, a jack the lad. Now he was grey: grey hair, grey skin, grey teeth, and grey eyes.

Then he didn't feel too clever. The hospital tests confirmed that it was back. The doctor said that nowadays, people live with cancer rather than die of it. Lee's type was aggressive, so we were to "remain hopeful but put your affairs in order." One-Nerve was crushed.

The whole gang was silent in front of Lee but chattered nonstop when he wasn't around. At first, it felt like we had all panicked, but then we all became incredibly calm and serious, as if we were mourning his passing before he had even gone.

We thought we might have a holiday before the treatments had to start. We got our matching daisies tattooed on the inside of our left wrists, booked a lovely B&B in Dorset, and then ... COVID hit.

And The World stopped.

I became Lee's full-time carer. It was so lonely and so scary. I had to take full responsibility for his safety and my own. I became obsessed with cleaning every surface, including our online shopping bags. I'd thoroughly bleach-wipe everything before it came into the house. I rearranged the furniture so we could stockpile all his boxes of drugs in the front room.

Lee could barely walk, but I made sure he sat outside in our garden for an hour a day. We talked and talked, but he was losing hope and then became irritable. He'd apologise when he said harsh things that were unfair, but he was so frustrated. He felt sorry for himself, and nothing interested him. His mates couldn't call in. Phone calls tired him. Zoom was even worse as he saw himself on camera and couldn't handle it.

"I already look like I've been dug up, Fi."

We had each other, but we were both so lonely.

Eventually, he said, "I just want to go, Fi."

We planned his funeral and thanked God for One-Nerve's wise head. His decision to take out life assurance all those years ago, when they first went into partnership, was paying off. If it had been up to me and Lee, we would never have thought to do this. We were both live-in-the-moment people. Stabbing-Nigel came up with the idea originally, and One-Nerve, for once, had listened to him.

The funeral song selection made us smile briefly. 'Dumb Ways to Die' by Tangerine Kitty seemed appropriate for a sparky, and 'Lily the Pink, with her Medicinal Compounds' by The Scaffold seemed appropriate for the chemo. We had visions of the mourners leaving the ceremony forced to be jolly while singing Lily the Pink, but of course, little did we know at the time, with Covid, that wouldn't happen.

Lee was giving up. He was grumpy every day, and if I asked what I could do for him, he got even grumpier. He would lash out and then say "Sorry" as he knew it wasn't my fault. But even his Sorrys were getting fewer. I got a little brass bell from my aunty, who thought it would come in useful if Lee needed anything and I was not in his room. I hated that bloody bell. I would sort him out, but just as I got back into the kitchen to start my breakfast, the bell would go off. We came up with a system: one ring, not urgent; it can wait 10 minutes, two rings, he needed to go to the loo, three rings, he'd wet himself. The incontinence was winning.

They gave us huge incontinence pants so he could go through the night, but the number of times I had to change him was unbelievable. Wet nappies were bearable, but the poo nappies were disgusting. I gagged but just had to get on with it.

One day, I made a huge mistake. He asked me what would be the first thing I would do with my Charlies Angels, "after both he and Covid had gone." I said, "I don't want to think about life without you," but he said, "Fi, I don't want to be here anymore. I'm done. I want to go," I screamed at him, "You ungrateful bastard, you can't just exit and leave me alone." We cried and hugged, but to be honest, the skeleton in the bed repulsed me; he had a sickly smell too. This figure wasn't the Lee I knew.

One day he said, "Have a smoke with me." I said gently, "No, it was hard giving it up."

"Come on, one last wish from a dying man."

Day after day he kept asking the same thing.

And I kept saying no, so he kept pleading.

"I don't want to go backwards," I said firmly.

"That's right, you selfish cow!" he snapped, "Because you've got a future."

There was no comeback; I swallowed hard and walked away.

The next time he was nasty again, I said, "Actually, I've been thinking about what I'd do when you're gone. I might do a para-chute jump." Then, quick as a flash, he said, "Careful, do they make parachutes that big; let's be real, darlin, you'll drop like a stone."

I stood up. I'd just changed him. He looked at me and smiled, a sly smile. And then the smell hit me.

"Not another fucking poo!" I screamed.

Then I couldn't help myself. I said, "Right, that's enough. You can just bloody well sit in it." So I walked past him and pushed the bell just out of his reach. I had to get out of the house. I rang the helpline, "Macmillan, it's time."

I told them that I couldn't do this anymore. I was near to break-ing point. The person at the other end of the helpline was brilliant. Lee would go to the hospice for respite—just a couple of weeks to give me a break. I was staring at his window, our home that I didn't want to go back into, and simply said, "Thank you," hung up, and then burst into tears.

Lee wasn't surprised when I told him; he nodded when I said I needed a break. So it was only going to be temporary. But we both knew it would be touch-and-go if he made it back home. He was disintegrating fast.

I saw him into the ambulance, told him I loved him and that I'd see him soon. He waved and said, "Left hand, my pocket rocket, daisy to daisy."

I waved, just not with the daisy hand. Back in the house, I felt numb and stared into space, not putting any lights on, even when it got dark. I had the best night's sleep in months.

The funeral was wrong. It was way too small for such a large character. Lee would have hated it. There was no fun in the readings; they were all serious. I kept thinking about our bar code on his left-toe joke because it would have been more appropriate than the daisies now. It was even more surreal with a video link for all his mates. It did feel like his body was just being dispatched. I was very miserable, but I had no tears. I was all cried out. The rest of our gang was wet enough. They all looked stunned. Molly was stuck in France and felt helpless, probably for the best. I could never deal with her hysteria at the best of times. She was Daddy's girl, so it would take her a while to accept his passing.

Everyone wanted to come round, but with Covid still running amok, I was quite happy to be alone.

The paperwork was a pain, and I left it to One-Nerve, Stabbing, and the solicitors. Their accountants raised a few eyebrows at the petrol station bills with more Ginsters than our local factory.

I had a big clear out, got rid of all the boxes of drugs, his bed, and the piles of incontinent pads. It was such a waste, but I understood with Covid that nothing could be recycled.

Six months went by, and I was still waiting for my grief counselling. Everyone was booked solid. I painted our bedroom and made it mine. I quite liked being alone, which surprised me as I had never been. Lee and I loved being sociable.

I was getting by on benefits until Lee's life assurance payout. Then Leanne suggested taking in a lodger to help with the bills and to keep me company. At first, I didn't like the idea, I didn't need company, but Leanne knew a mature student who was going to the local college and needed digs. She would be no trouble and would keep out of my way.

I agreed, so Agnes from Bulgaria arrived. She was clean, a bit hard to understand, and very serious. She kept herself to herself.

One night, I offered Agnes a glass of wine. After our second glass, she told me she'd just broken up with her boyfriend. She met online. He sounded like a real creep. He'd been stringing her along with two other women, and when she called him out on it, he made her feel stupid. Another glass of wine, with more stories, and we were howling with laughter. I couldn't remember the last time I'd laughed this hard. I told her I'd heard a bit about online dating, but it sounded like something the kids could deal with more than someone my age. I knew about false promises, out-of-date photos, catfishing scams, and ghosting. It wasn't for me. Anyway, I wasn't ready to get back out there; too soon.

She asked me how old I was. I told her, "fifty-eight."

She said, "That's ok, you not ready. But still young. Young enough for love. Old men want younger woman to take care for them."

"Sod that!" I said, "I don't want to be anyone's carer ever again."

"You can be cougar – maybe fifteen years younger, no strings?"

"No, that's not my thing. One day, maybe another Lee, my age, though."

"So, time for blue pills."

"What's that?"

"Viagra for him," and then she makes the action of a tampon being put in, "and slippery pills for you. You need help." And then, in broken English, she wags her finger, saying, "Remember, don't use it, you lose it. No pill for you. Ouch!"

I'd heard a bit about this, but not enough. I must have been so distracted. Have I written myself off? Is it too late?

"I'm not ready for that yet, but I'll tell you what I am ready for... a tattoo on my right wrist."

| 5 |

Voices in your head.

Welcome back. This podcast is not to be taken lightly.

It will blow your mind!

Let's start with a couple of statistics.

According to the Gov.UK 'Prescribed Medicines Review,' 7.3 million adults (17%) were prescribed antidepressants.

Prescriptions for women were 1.5 times higher than those for men, and these rates generally increase with age.

In a study of more than 1,000 women aged 50+, in addition to the physical symptoms of menopause, 62% experienced mood-related symptoms, and 31% reported mental health issues.

And, of course, the aftermath of Covid will drive these figures higher still because where there is a chronic illness, there is mental stress too.

Looking more closely at the data from a mental health study in England, we found startling peaks for women at 16-24 years and 45-54 years.

What are the factors driving these peaks? What is going on? Does what troubled us in our youth come back and bite us later on? Hold on to that thought.

No mistaking it, mental health is on the agenda now, loud and clear, as is menopause.

These are *big* topics. So let's join the dots.

I'm going to be flying solo on this podcast. Whilst I am not a mental health expert, I, too, have moments of doubt, moments of sadness, and moments of worry. I'm sure everything will be fine, but will it?

Women are good at juggling. It is what we do; it's what we've always done.

So why does it feel harder now? Well, we're getting older, maybe wiser, and the challenges at this stage of our lives are serious: empty nest, ageing parents, health and relationship concerns, and all this against the backdrop of a society that values youth.

When did we start losing the plot?

Many of us are unprepared for menopause, blindly going through the routines of our lives before the awareness happens: weight gain by stealth, patchy periods, and the erosion of our sleep window. These symptoms creep up in the perimenopause phase. The penny drops when three or more collide. As the saying goes, one symptom is a fluke, two is a coincidence, but three is a trend we shouldn't ignore.

And that is only half of the equation because as physical symptoms present, so too come the mental ones: the vague and errant brain, the zero to sixty, sweet to sour mood swings, and from absolute certainty to crippling self-doubt.

When others see glimpses of the turmoil that's going on inside, normal is no longer normal. Loved ones may function as our pressure valves, but sometimes even they do not know our sense of overwhelm. So when is it time to call in the professionals?

We all have random thoughts, conversations, and criticisms that may never leave the safety of our heads. How they interplay with our daily lives can be a help or a hindrance.

Let's meet these voices in our heads. The inner coach – let's think of that voice as the angel and the inner critic – well, that makes this the demon. One lifts us, and one trips us up. Our inner voice (the Self) is unfettered and unfiltered. In any scenario, there will always be the spoken voices, sometimes moderated, but nevertheless the main tool for interpersonal communication.

Rarely do we speak our mind.

As life events unfold, ask yourself, whose voice is the loudest?

A typical domestic scenario – children, laundry, and roast dinner discoveries.

she says: *"lunch will be ready in 30 mins guys"*

the know-it-all: "have you washed my sports kit yet?"

she thinks: wonder what Lycra would look like on the ABBA girls now.

the know-it-all (sees confusion): "hello, anyone in there?" (waving arms frantically)

she thinks: listen smart arse, next time, do your own washing

she says: *"watch it, clever clogs; it's in the dryer"*

the sulky one: "if you've done his, when's mine being washed?"

she thinks: for f***s sake, that's another load!

demon: just shake it and fold it; they'll never know

angel: you wouldn't do that

she says: *"I'll do that load after lunch"*

demon: tick tock, the clock's ticking on that lunch

angel: delegate

she says: *"please put the cauliflower cheese into the oven"*

noisy dog: yap, yap, yap (while running off with a school shoe)

she says: *"grab that shoe!"*

demon: don't bother; I see you haven't polished it yet

angel: another chore to delegate

the sulky one: "what the hell is this?"

(Presents a dish of unrecognisable carbon)

she says: "oi Language!"

demon: you've done it again

she thinks: shut up, you sarcastic twit, the house is still standing, and no one is hurt

the sulky one: "Is that the leeks in cheese sauce from last week?"

she thinks: Oh SHIT!

Lady X is in perimenopause and has only recently started to experience low levels of anxiety and mental exhaustion. These present as bouts of forgetfulness and decreases in concentration. In her late teens, she had minor episodes of anxiety. With strong friendship groups and activities that she excelled in, Lady X could ride the hormonal rollercoaster successfully. Her pregnancies were uplifting but uneventful, and she didn't suffer the baby blues with the births of any of her children. Her mother was discreet like the rest of that generation, leaving her unprepared for the menopause. She has a keen sense of self.

"I have my moments, but on the whole, I'm feeling fine."

Let's look at another typical social scenario – best friend's second wedding reception, Lady Y is without a partner.

demon: you need a drink

she says: "I'll have a glass of fizz, please. In fact I'll take two, thank you."

demon: down them both; it'll calm you

angel: sip slowly, stay in control.

demon: someone's coming over, friend or foe?

(host makes introductions)

she says: "oh dear, I'm never going to remember your names"

angel: just keep smiling

demon: with that grimace; who cares, you'll never see them again anyway

angel: your heart's racing; stay calm; you've got this

demon: Palpitations! At your age? Is there a doctor in the room?

she thinks: oh, shut up

angel: never mind your age, take a deep breath; you look amazing

demon: yes, amazingly well preserved, as in formaldehyde.

(confiding to her friend)

she says: "I feel old, I feel uncomfortable, I just don't belong."

(later, waiting at the bar, younger women are being served first)

she thinks: Wow! When did I lose my impact?

demon: that's because you've become invisible!

(barman spills a drink on her)

barman says: "sorry, love, didn't see you there"

she says: "Oh SHIT!"

Lady Y is menopausal. She's had a low mood for some time. Her early hormonal years were reasonably uneventful, apart from periods of anxiety when her generous shape did not fit the norm of the time. The only other occasion she felt she was not herself was with the baby blues after her first child.

Now her new menopausal body has lowered her self-esteem. She feels this shape has associated health risks; a recent health check confirmed this. Her acute anxiety levels can lead to panic attacks, often leaving her with a sense of dread. To top it all off, she recently lost her partner and feels lonely.

"I'm not myself; the panics come out of the blue and make me feel like I can't breathe."

Final scenario – business meeting; Lady Z, looking flustered, arrives late.

she says: *"email crisis, it had to be done"*

demon: really? You should have left it till after the meeting

angel: but you made sure that it was perfect

she thinks: this meeting is such a waste of my time

she says: *"do I really need to be here?"*

boss says: "yes, you do!"

demon: I'd fire the lot of them,

angel: but you can't do this on your own.

(Agenda item: Project deadline brought forward)

she says: *"where the hell did that come from?"*

a colleague says: "that was your suggestion last meeting I believe"

demon: guess that one dropped off your list too, shame

angel: think smart, don't react

she says: *"alright, smart arse. It's all in hand*

she thinks: Christ Almighty!

boss says: "new deadlines, non-negotiable, end of!"

demon: Reload. Aim. Fire!

she says: *"I guess we don't have a choice then!"*

boss says: "moving on; we haven't got all morning"

she thinks: that's me swamped, then

demon: go on, give them both barrels

she says: *"quite, as you've f***ing wasted most of it!"*

angel: ouch

she thinks: SHIT, SHIT, SHIT!

Lady Z is postmenopausal. She's become increasingly irritable and sharp since perimenopause. Her moods are frustrating her, as well as the nearest and dearest people in her life. As a child, she was always the daydreamer and felt the odd one out. She is bright and creative but felt that her experimental behaviour labelled her as a problem teen. She admits to still regularly chasing the 'highs.' However, her success has always come at a price. Her brilliance is recognised, but her erratic behaviour makes her a loose cannon. Her postnatal depression was severe and damaged many relationships. This is the worst she's ever felt, and she has a crippling sense of shame.

"Bloody hell, how many people do I need to murder to get help?"

To summarise.

Three women: three typical scenarios, three different mental states, and three menopausal stages. They are all in need of a different approach to care. Their journeys through life and menopause are as individual as they are.

It's taken a while for **Lady X** to recognise that menopause has started. First, she put her patchy periods down to stress. Then, it took two or more symptoms on top of that for her to realise that it had arrived.

Her scenario paints a picture of a woman in a safe, unguarded home environment. Her voices are merely distractions. She still has a sense of self and is outwardly calm. But should we be able to look into the future at Lady X in a different menopausal stage, after a changing life event, who knows what those voices could sound like and which one would be the loudest? Would she still be in control? She won't know until she gets there.

At present, her score on the **Menopause Rating Scale (MRS) – psychological subscale is 5/16,** which puts her into the mild category. However, her lifestyle supports a healthy mental state, so she doesn't need any intervention currently but will keep it under review.

So if that's considered 'normal' or depending on the nature of her mental health expression, experts may say, 'Neurotypical', where are you sitting? Let's step it up a bit.

Lady Y is vastly different. She's vocalising that she feels unheard, unseen, and generally written off. In her scenario, her loudest voice is the demon, her critic. Maybe that demon represents a voice from her past. She was once vital and felt it. What's happened? Why has she lost her confidence? She's critical about her out-of-shape body. Her critical eye triggers her emotional distress, anxiety, and depression. Her disordered eating has been a cyclical trap. She's wearing vulnerability with her mood and body language, yet other women with similar shapes consider themselves vital and sexy. And guess what? They are; they own it. Once Lady Y recognises that she needs help to break the cycle, it's a step towards self-investment.

Her **MRS psychological sub scale is 9/16,** which puts her in the moderate category.

I know this woman; I hold her close to me. She needs to see what I see and believe she's worthy; she is enough.

Lady Z is in a different league of distress entirely. She's already realised her symptoms have evolved over the years, and now that she's in post-menopause, she fears that her inner restlessness and inattention are escalating. She's still working but worries that her performance is below par and her extra hours to keep up are exhausting her. She says, "It's not fair; just as I'm at the top of my game, my body and mind have betrayed me."

At the time of the test, Lady Z's **MRS psychological subscale is 14/16,** putting her in the severe category.

Let's face it, with that score, it's off to the professionals she should go.

What moves these three narratives: of mild, moderate, and severe, from general menopausal symptoms to common mental health expressions or disorders?

And when are you considered profoundly affected, possibly a danger to self and others?

These three ladies will be having different conversations with any medical expert should they seek help from the professionals.

We don't need to read a headline to know that many women suffer in silence. Thank goodness that menopause is on the table, but society is still playing catch up. For many women, the stigma of menopause is felt mainly in the workplace.

Let's take a moment to digest this.

Which stigma? Being a woman? Being a menopausal woman? Constantly having to work harder and smarter simply to catch up.

We are already fighting every label and cliché that comes our way while discretely managing a natural, cognitive, and biological transition. So let's be clear this is not a disease.

Surely we deserve respect and support, especially as society's fastest-growing economically active segment.

The only thing that has changed is that our oestrogen is in decline. This decline and what it means may explain the movement towards relaxing the accessibility to hormone replacement therapy. Again, think of the cost implications here. Productivity costs, long-term health costs: these are big numbers.

Another consideration is that three different journeys are running parallel here: ageing, menopause, and our genetic predisposition. All of these carry psychological flags that may interweave along these parallels. As a result, stress, anxiety, and depression, along with sleep problems and mood swings, lurk beneath the surface, compounded by societal and environmental exposure levels.

While we carry the protective shield that's oestrogen, mental distress tends to be regulated. However, that doesn't mean life events coupled with emotional stressors can't aggravate our mental state; the reactions may differ across individuals.

Does it matter how we classify these? Depression is depression, right? Not quite. Of course, it matters which path you attribute these symptoms to. The more specific the diagnosis, the more precise the treatments can be. Anti-anxiety pills are different from antidepressants. Anti-psychotic drugs offer another form of targeted therapy. And HRT, well, that targets reproductive hormone imbalances.

Earlier, when I asked you to hold that thought as you reflected on the hormonal stages of your life, this is where it's led us to.

In puberty, the surge of sex hormones plays havoc with our body and brain. It's a physically and mentally turbulent time for us.

Postpartum depression, with its significant decrease in oestrogen, may have also contributed to a decline in mental health. Studies indicate that oestrogen has been known to mask pre-existing mental illness, perhaps up to now, undiagnosed. Now in menopause, mental health symptoms may be amplified.

How this hormonal cocktail, with its highs and lows, played out *in puberty and postpartum* may play out *now in our menopause*.

I like to think of it as riding the oestrogen wave.

Armed with what we've covered, let's imagine the questions our ladies may use in consultation with a medical professional.

Lady X

Her mental health symptoms are minor. She manages her moods with supplements and lifestyle. She's reluctant to consider HRT because of the mixed messages about its safety. She carries a low-level risk factor. She may seek over-the-counter HRT offerings if her symptoms disrupt her quality of life.

Lady Y

Her mood continues to sink; she knows from her past that she's prone to depression. Her previous mental health incidents have always resulted in antidepressants with side effects of sexual dysfunction and weight gain. Her recent health checks have confirmed that chronic illnesses could be on the horizon. First her mental health, now her physical health. The wheels are beginning to fall off. Where should she start?

Frequent appointments with her GP and lack of specialist knowledge have made her feel unsupported.

She's always thinking, "I don't care how much you know until I know how much you care."

Let's not leave Lady Y waiting; let's give her a dream consultation without time pressure.

The GP brings up her medical history, which includes the mental health episodes, treatments, and how she felt at each stage of *her* oestrogen wave.

They discuss her current symptoms with her recent MRS rating score on each subscale. Her history and the increasing frequency of her sense of panic, they agree that she needs to see a specialist.

With the psychological subscale, the specialists will explore further the context of her sense of self, her outward behaviour in social settings, and the stress level this causes her. Who is behind that critical 'voice' in her head? Past or present, alive or dead? She may need a support team behind her. If prescription drugs are an option, then she needs to ask:

Why this particular drug?

What are the options?

What are the risks?

What are the side effects?

When do we revisit the timeline? (Some medication loses efficacy as you age.)

The moral of her story is:

Ladies, take responsibility. Whether you have an excellent GP, a visiting intern, or a misdiagnosis from the past, the health service remains under pressure. Your diagnosis, your treatment plan. Actively take part. Own it.

Lady Z

Remember her? You'll agree that her story sets her apart from the others. Her worsening cognitive symptoms of memory impairment and difficulties with planning and organisation led to her visit with her GP. After a referral to a specialist, she has since been diagnosed with ADHD. It's just one of a handful of specific neurodiversity's that women have recently been diagnosed with. So whether you have been recognised as having High Sensitivity or Sensory Processing Disorder (SPD); or have been given a diagnosis of Autism or ADHD; these neurological expressions need specialist intervention and care, and quite probably a range of blended treatments.

She always knew she was different but was undiagnosed until now. She will always wonder if diagnosis and treatment had come earlier, how different her life may have played out, especially with her postpartum oestrogen plummets. After finally being diagnosed, she feels liberated with newfound self-acceptance.

Just remember, 'Prescription without proper diagnosis is malpractice.'

Let's work together and make sure that we get it right.

We've come a long way. Things are going in the right direction. Mental health is firmly on the agenda, and the impact of menopause on our workforce is registered. So whether you present as neurotypical or neurodiverse, you may still experience anxiety and depression. We need an accurate identification because the more we understand neurodiversity, refine the treatments available, the more society will be able to accept and retain valuable and vital women. The future is looking brighter.

I've said I was flying solo on this one; now, let's land this topic.

Mind blown yet?

Well, try this. In 1900 the average age for menopause was 48 years. A woman's life expectancy at that time was also 48 years. Our current life expectancy is around 87 years, meaning we still have a third of our life left. We deserve to live it well and believe in the power of the human spirit.

I'm going to leave you with these three points:

1. Know yourself and your life's journey.
2. Work with the professionals if necessary and actively partici-pate in any diagnosis.
3. Choose your options wisely.

My final thought.

Menopausal women are not mad, but if you patronise or fob us off, we will become f***ing furious.

Join us next time as we hear women's views about ageing around the globe.

| 6 |

Charlie's story

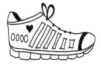

It's her voice, the voice from my past. The same soothing tones and inflexions, the same sexy, smoky undertone, but mostly, the voice that caresses and rebukes in equal measures. Cara, my obsession, my saviour, and my tormentor. With one call, my past collides with my present.

"Darling, how are you? Where've you been all my life? I've missed you, Charlie."

"Be careful what you desire," she used to say. How ironic then that this is the call I've waited, no longed for, for nearly half my life, and yet here I am, clutching the phone, heart pounding and wishing that I hadn't pressed that green button.

Do you know the cliche: it takes two to tango? Well, that wasn't entirely true with Cara. She tangoed while I was swept up in her perfumed embrace, struggling to keep pace and getting hopelessly lost in the rhythm. Three years that lasted. Oh, there were many times I walked away, or perhaps if I'm honest, I was discarded like a used condom. But like the proverbial moth to the flame, I kept

80

getting drawn back into her hedonistic world. But, again, I'll add, in the spirit of honesty, dear reader; I willingly gave in. She was tall, dark, and incredibly sensual. I lost my mind to her. I lost myself in her repeatedly. She was the perfect seducer, and I, the unknowing victim.

"Darling, I must see you. I want to look into those beautiful dark eyes of yours again."

Every word she utters is like a mini explosion. I struggle to hear her as my thoughts race back and forth in time, my heart contracting with emotion. For God's sake, Charlie, get a grip.

Like most people, I navigate life's difficulties with a careful, considered approach. That's not to say I'm impervious to the blows that can come my way. I can usually pick myself up, dust myself off and move forward with a new resolve. Oh, there have been a few devastating events that threatened to derail me, yet somehow, I've survived. Cara was one such event. She came into my life when I needed validation. I was vulnerable, questioning my choices. That period with her gave me a sense of belonging. How deluded I was. But let me not get ahead of myself; perhaps I should start at the beginning. A story that begins in my childhood.

When I was four, my parents dressed me in a sailor suit for my birthday. This memory is so clear, the little white suit with its white and blue trimmed hat to match. My young self, appraising the serious little sailor staring back at me in the mirror. Oh, the feeling this memory invokes, still to this day. Finally, I felt seen. You might be asking, what can that mean to a four-year-old? Well, I can't be any clearer than that. A recognition of who I truly was, is what it felt like. My father was in the navy at the time. The structure and discipline that it gave him were evident in his deportment. He took such pride in his appearance. This scaled-down outfit made me stand taller and prouder too. It gave me the same sense of belonging, his and now mine. That moment, that feeling, never leaves me.

According to my mother, I also spilt cherry red cordial down the front of that suit, yet I have no lasting memories related to that.

By and large, I had a happy childhood. All felt Father's absences, but I always felt safe and cocooned with loving grandparents to step in and assist where necessary. I was a quiet child, well-behaved, and always willing to help. School provided an opportunity to make friends, but it was the company of teachers I sought. As an only child, I enjoyed their attention. I liked that I could hold the floor with my impressive knowledge of British naval history. Unfortunately, my quirky nature, while precocious to grownups, also made me a target for the bullies among my peers. In our little village school, being different was not good.

"Charlie was a quiet but confident child. She worked hard and seemed to get on with everyone. Didn't have many friends, though."

Father's first posting abroad shook my world. This time Mother and I were to accompany him. I was ten when we moved to the Middle East. This move triggered so many emotions for us. Mother was excited to experience the expatriate lifestyle, while Father was relieved at having his family close. I felt somewhat betrayed by their decision. We were leaving our picture postcard English country cottage with its proximity to my grandparents. It took much convincing and a new bike thrown in for good measure to forgive them for this major upheaval. It wasn't long before I was beguiled by the uniqueness of it all. This strange but exotic country was a melting pot of different nationalities and ethnicities. As expats in the naval compound, we found ourselves settling into the rhythms of this community. Mother was expected to dress modestly, but as a child, I had more freedom. Thanks to my father's complexion, I was soon nut brown and enjoying the outdoor life. Despite the heat, sports consumed our time.

"What an active bunny Charlie was. Her passion for running started then. She never complained about the heat. You should see the medals we've accumulated over the years. Tennis, hockey, track events; you name it, Charlie earned it."

Running with Father was a special bonding experience. It was always hard for me when he was away at sea. Any time spent with him felt precious. He had so many exciting stories to share. I enjoyed the quiet time we spent together. On the other hand, Mother was very social and constantly included me in her ever-growing circle of friends.

"When Charlie was my tennis partner, we were unbeatable; an elite player. So seeing the look on their faces when she arrived dressed in her tennis gear was funny. Priceless!"

School was uneventful; friends came and went. This transient ex-pat life made me aware of how easily people come into your lives, some with meaning and purpose. Unfortunately, they leave just as easily. A stable home life and happily married parents provided the balance I needed. Back then, I was never any good at adapting to change. Stability mattered to me then, and it does so now. Sometimes it feels like it's taken a lifetime to discover this. Demanding? No. Discerning? Maybe.

I was never fussy with food, though, eating most things. The many types of cuisines reflected the multi-cultural society we were part of. Many households, like ours, could afford to have staff. We had an Asian helper who used to clean and cook on occasion. Her love of spice and her skill at making delicious curries opened my eyes and awakened my tastebuds to non-British food. She used to laugh at my insistence that dosa breakfast pancakes had to be smothered with cinnamon sugar and lemon, not chickpea and lentil curry. Nevertheless, I enjoyed trying new flavour combinations.

For the next few years, this life was idyllic. Almost too good to be true. But change was inevitable. The combination of my age and another post for my father meant they decided to send me back to a boarding school in England. While this news was heart-breaking for us all, the steadfastness of my father and his assurances that this was character-building made me determined not to show any emotion and to accept my fate.

"Smooth seas don't make skilful sailors," he was fond of saying when times were tough.

That move to boarding school felt like I was starting all over again. I had extended family in the next county, my safety net, and although the first few weeks in this unfamiliar environment were rough, I knew I had an escape route. After a while, I enjoyed the regimented lifestyle, not so much the people. Lessons were hard, and the teachers were strict, but I persevered. My flavour palate changed, in fact, drastically reduced, and suddenly meal choices were restricted to a two-week menu. Gone were the eye-watering Eastern curries, the spicy sauces, and the creamy, fruity drinks to soothe the tongue. Though wholesome and adequate, school dinners lacked the flavour I'd learned was possible.

It was during one of these mealtimes in the cafeteria that I met Anya. She caught me rolling my eyes as I placed some mushy vegetables on my plate, and she smiled knowingly. Our lament at the blandness of the meals and our shared love of spicy Indian curries meant we were always sneaking off at weekends to scavenge. We always looked for the sweetest, the tartest, or the spiciest morsels. She was so knowledgeable about spices and flavours and, already at that age, was a great cook. Her family were adventurous eaters, and the occasional weekend visits to her home took me on gastronomic adventures.

Anya was everything I was not, socially and emotionally. She was exceedingly popular and quick to make friends, while I usually hung back and waited to be included. Her feisty nature and her competitive spirit made her good at sports, and it was on the hockey field that our friendship continued to grow. I couldn't help admiring her changing body as I became aware of my scrawny own.

Anya developed quickly, and her curvy body soon became the envy of the other girls and turned many a boy's head when we were out in town. But it was my eye she sought in a crowd, my hand she grabbed and held to her bosom when she was excited, and my shoulder she rested her head on when she was tired. After a while, this closeness took on a different meaning as we began exploring each other's bodies in the dark, not making too much noise for fear of being caught. Those forbidden kisses and tentative touches ignited feelings in me that were new and exciting. We'd opened a Pandora's box, and there was no going back. So many rumours were going around at the time. After all, we were at a girls' boarding school, with a gropy prefect here and a lecherous teacher there. Still, what we secretly did felt shameful, but somehow it felt right. I thought I loved her and told her so many, many times.

She laughed, teased, and said, "We are young; our lives lay ahead of us. Our coupling means nothing; it's just a fun way to pass the time." She used to joke, "We will be each other's bridesmaids, marry our professional men, have many babies, and grow fat and happy."

But I knew deep down this was not my fate.

For a long time, our discretion paid off, but it was on a weekend visit to her home that her brother caught us, thereby finally exposing our night-time activities. Her parents were devastated and threatened to tell mine, but in the end, they didn't. Even after promising them we would no longer see each other; they moved Anya to a different college to complete her A-levels. I was devastated. My sadness didn't go unnoticed by my family, but I couldn't bring myself to tell them about Anya, about me, not yet. Their assumption that I was nursing a broken heart was correct, not that I'd "get over it and meet another boy." I had watched Anya pack her things and leave; her goodbye was fleeting. After that, I vowed never to let anyone into my heart again.

My university offers put me at a crossroads again. It was tempting to follow a military or naval path; the pressure was there. But it was a business degree that called me in the end. My dating life was almost non-existent during this time. Two very academic years passed by quickly. I didn't envy the prolific social lives of my classmates. On the contrary, I welcomed the library's silence: my refuge, my solace. In my last year, I flat shared with three other students who have since become good friends.

"Charlie always seemed so sad and lonely. She was never interested in meeting anyone. She didn't talk about her love life then."

I still carried so much heartache and hurt from my school years. As a result, I wasn't interested in getting to know anyone else. I preferred being alone, and people stopped asking me why after a while.

"Charlie had the most extensive spice collection, more so than anyone else; it was never going to be just salt and pepper when she cooked."

I still loved cooking and was happy to take over this duty in our flat share.

"Parties in our flat were legendary. Charlie made sure of that. She cooked the most delicious meals, even on a student budget."

My meals were far from the ordinary. I knew how to add flavour to food. And where to shop, even with my limited budget.

"She was always so meticulous, a bit scary to live with, to be honest. Her room was always spotless, and she didn't take kindly to us when we were messy, which often happened!"

Shared living was a challenge, my flatmates were messy, and I told them so on many occasions.

Romantic interest during this time? Again too complicated. Friends quickly worked out my preferences. Near the end of my final year, I started dating again. Friends usually set up blind dates. Some were interesting enough to warrant a second date; others were disasters. I recall one date whose face and body had so many piercings that I was too afraid to kiss her for fear of things getting caught. No relationships for me then, just sometimes casual sex. After graduation, I moved to London, and my foray into the publishing world coincided with my entrance onto the gay scene. This new life felt liberating after keeping myself to myself for so long. Work socials and the many clubs and bars gave me plenty of fodder, and I'm not ashamed to say that I lost control for a while. Music, drugs, and the punk rock scene were intoxicating, but it wasn't long before Aids made itself known. As with most young people, you think it will never happen to you until it does—only not me, but a good friend. The GAY cancer, that's what they called it. It felt like a real threat; we felt vulnerable. The shockwaves this death sent into my newfound community made me decide to come out to my family finally. It took a family weekend away and being propped up by a bottle of red wine before I finally found the courage to say those loaded words. "I'm gay."

It was my father's face I watched closely. Mother always encouraged me to be different and follow my path, so I knew she would accept it. Father, as I suspected he would, needed time. It took a few months for my father to acknowledge this facet of my life. His strict, conservative upbringing and naval background had shaped his outlook. While our radio silence was unfathomable, he had to come to terms with my disclosure in his way. My lifestyle choice and the trials I'd face were difficult for him to accept. At a time when 'being gay' meant being a social outcast, his concern was that I would find it impossible to assimilate. My path would always be difficult, and he felt powerless to assist. It took a lifelong dream of his and our shared love of running, for him to sign us up for the London marathon. He hoped that the task of training for and completing this colossal challenge would set me up for whatever hardships awaited me. And he knew there'd be plenty. His triumph, my achievement, was glorious. It also was my first lesson in perseverance.

My past showed me that my emotional state could be fragile. Future relationships may hang in the balance, but it's worth putting yourself out there. To always be open to new possibilities.

Then, almost as if she were summoned, I met Cara.

She was forty-two to my twenty-seven but looked ten years younger. She epitomised style and elegance as only the French can do. She was also loaded, a combination of a trust fund and a wealthy ex-husband. She lived large, throwing lavish dinner parties and was often spotted clubbing with the young, the glamorous, and the rich and famous. Our worlds collided at one of her famous soirees. I wasn't meant to be there. A late invitation was issued when the beauty editor at the publishing house asked me to accompany her. Her date had cancelled at the last minute. My newfound confidence, a killer body, having just trained for and run a marathon, and a borrowed leather catsuit to match a 'come as you dare' theme, placed me directly in the sights of this huntress. Initially, she was interested in my experiences in the Middle East, my job, and the clubs I frequented. As time wore on, she pursued me relentlessly—flowers to my workplace, chance meetings at work socials, and long-drawn-out telephone calls. I was slowly succumbing. Finally, I agreed to go out with her. Champagne, oysters, and dimly lit restaurants were among the many tools of her seductive trade. Oh she knew what she was doing. By the end of the evening, I was begging her to take me to bed.

"Darling, tell me how much you desire me. Tell me how much you want to fuck me."

What followed was the most turbulent three years of my life. Power corrupts, they say. It was true for her, for me. Cocaine-fuelled parties were closely followed by writhing bodies on sweat-soaked sheets: her body, my body, anybody. Our goddess, Cara, rose like a phoenix out of the smoky, ashy detritus of our wild nights. Ready to start the cycle all over again. When we dared to fan the flames of her narcissistic behaviour, we were banished from her bedroom, home, and life.

Why did I keep going back, you ask? Wouldn't you? So many guilty pleasures and the feeling of being untethered, liberated in her hedonistic world.

Cara was impossible to refuse, and her world of opulence and excess was even harder to resist. I longed to be a part of it all. Her guests and her friends; so talented, worldly and privileged. To continue participating in those long, drawn-out dinner table discussions about life's meaning, purpose, and futility. Gliding effortlessly through this sumptuous world of drugs, art, fine dining, and travel to exotic places. We holidayed in St Tropez in the summer and skied in Courchevel in the winter. I was seduced on so many levels. And the sex, the mind-blowing sex that was always there for the taking. I wanted to remain a part of it all. I wanted to be her, to be with her.

It took a lot of courage to say those words to Cara finally. In her world, love was such an alien concept.

"Love, what do you mean, love? That's for the weak, the pathetic. I worship beautiful sexy bodies, darling. That's all that matters, fucking beautiful bodies."

I wanted so much more with her, from her. I wanted her to feel the tenderness and permanence that a deep and meaningful relationship offered.

"Darling, you mean nothing to me. Girls like you are everywhere, ripe for the taking."

My loving pleas were ignored. Brutal words continued to spill forth from her lips.

"Stop that pitiful crying, darling; it's not a good look on you."

Yes, I wept. And begged and pleaded with Cara. After three years of satisfying her every need, I was no longer desirable in her eyes, savagely discarded. So what if I did want more? I needed to know that I was important to her. I wished for a stable life; I deserved love and respect from her, none of which she was willing to give. Every rejection was another wound in my heart. The final shock was flaunting her new, much younger lover at an event we'd both attended. My life, my world, it all came crashing down.

Everything I held dear up to that point had taken a back seat to my obsession with Cara. My family, quietly disapproving, so kept at a distance; my job, a financial necessity, yet meaningless; my running, a distraction, a waste of precious time, and so on.

I felt robbed of my youth and drained of my vitality. A dried-up husk at the age of thirty. As youngsters nowadays would so eloquently say, I had "literally lost my shit."

It left me believing that I wasn't worthy of love and that the happy ending that so many friends were finding was beyond my reach. My health suffered. I had no appetite and frequently skipped meals. Heartbreak took its toll on my body, my skin, my hair. Without my usual exercise fix, I failed to manage my mood and existed in a state of high anxiety and depression. Leaving my flat became laborious. It took every ounce of energy I could muster to go to work every day. It would provoke a panic attack if I thought I spotted Cara at work or in public. Life became unbearable. Friends propped me up as best they could. The usual "You'll get over her" and "Plenty of fish in the sea" didn't help. I felt lost.

In the end, "Mother knows best."

A friend's casual mention of Cara and her new paramour reduced me to floods of tears. All this happened while Mother was visiting. Intuitively she'd known that this relationship had been life-changing for me. Now faced with the reality of my loss and the grief I was experiencing; she knew that professional help was the only way to deal with it. To see me so emotionally broken, a shadow of my former self, was hard for her.

Nevertheless, she continued to be there for me with patience and sometimes harsh words, ensuring I ate balanced meals again. She also arranged for me to see someone. My psychotherapy sessions finally helped me understand my role as a victim in that toxic relationship. An epiphany was a further recognition of the predatory behaviours of my Svengali. My recovery was a lengthy and painful one. After two years, I still wasn't ready to start dating again. Throughout my ordeal, my work colleagues were incredibly supportive. I had managed to hold on to my job, only just. A change of scenery was recommended, so I moved into a more administrative role. I quickly realised that this suited me more. I discovered my love of running again and heeding sound advice, avoiding the pressure of races. Instead, I found the green spaces in the city and jogged my way around all the parks. This fresh perspective was very welcoming.

A few years later, I left my job in the city. Moving back in with my ageing parents was far from ideal, but a necessary temporary step. Their coastal home with direct access to the seafront and the promenade was refreshing, and it wasn't long before I felt confident enough to enter the local marathon. Father was close to retirement age but still in peak condition, so again joined me. On our training runs, he shared many stories of his life at sea. Our collective insights on all the exciting places we had visited are memories I continue to cherish. Between the huffing and puffing, we also shared our thoughts on the heartaches and the joys of life. I lost my father shortly after that. An unfortunate car accident brought an end to his retirement dream. This loss was profound, but this time I was better equipped to deal with it all. His wise words will forever stay with me.

It took a year and a few unsuccessful applications to find an administrative role in a South Downs secondary school. While the money didn't come close to my city salary, the opportunity to collaborate with a team in this countryside location was perfect.

I soon moved into a small flat nearby and welcomed my first rescue dog, Duke. Like me, he was still young but had a troubled past. He had the saddest eyes. At our first encounter, I fell in love with him when he shook his scrawny body and came tootling over to me as if to say, "Right, let's get on with it then." He became my furry running partner, and we flourished together. In time, I joined a running club and had a not-so-serious fling with one of the members. She knew I wasn't ready for emotional attachments and was happy to keep it casual.

Duke took no exception to this arrangement either and wasn't offended in the slightest that her little terrier cross would occasionally stay over. Dating with no emotional expectations was liberating. It provided many opportunities to explore the countryside together. We joined a hiking group and participated in walking challenges supporting animal rescue shelters. I enjoyed cooking meals for her. Our couplings, while tender, were merely an exchange of mutual pleasure, and we avoided saying anything we did not mean. I was happy for her when she met someone two years later and fell in love. The closure of this chapter was the catalyst to undertake a much-longed-for journey by myself finally. I was turning forty and decided to make this milestone birthday significant. I'd always wanted to visit India, and as a nod to my fathers heritage, that's what I did. I was drawn to the culture, the spices, and the people. They felt like my people. This solo journey fulfilled me in unexpected ways. The hustle and bustle of the city streets made me appreciate the peace and tranquillity of the countryside. I was moved by the plight of the impoverished and the many stray animals that roamed the streets. I learnt so much about the healing properties of Asian ingredients. By the end of my stay, I was spiritually ready for the week I'd booked into an Ashram. Here in this healing centre, I was introduced to meditation. Some of the rituals and chants learned here have become part of my everyday life.

"The power you have is to pause and be in the moment. To feel it, to know it, to learn from it."

Renewed vigour and an enlightened outlook are what I brought back with me into my job at school. It was at the start of the new term that I met Helen. She was the newest recruit, a PE and sports teacher. She seemed friendly and chatty with an infectious laugh.

By this time, I'd been working there for over five years. It felt like a lifetime. Our once ordinary, low-ranking school had blossomed into a highly rated school, and we were all enormously proud of our students. I was working in student admissions then, and although each passing year brought the same challenges and the same pressure, I enjoyed the predictability of the school year. I loved the high energy at the start of the term and the quenched depletion at the end in this ever-changing student environment with its firm but fair leadership.

"Charlie is calm under pressure and gets the job done. A delight to work with, but don't mess with her!"

I admit that I can be a bit difficult at times. I'm efficient because I care and I work to deadlines.

"Integral part of the team, can't do without her."

I love my job. I get on well with all the staff, and we often gather in the staff room to exchange funnies. Our students also keep us entertained with their teacher impersonations.

"Calls it as she sees it, so she's not always popular with the parents; that's okay though, keeps out the riffraff!"

It's the parents that make us all earn our keep. I don't take kindly to the chancers I encounter when processing admission applications. But I've learnt not to be intimidated by these types. Maybe a gift from my past.

From the start, staff and students alike were attracted to Helen. She was cheerful and charmed everyone with her easy manner and radiant smile. It didn't take her long to settle into her role in the team. Our chemistry wasn't instant, but I liked her and enjoyed her sense of humour. I'd heard she'd just been through a messy divorce through the staff grapevine. They'd only been married for two years. I'd also heard that she'd instigated it due to infidelity; on his part. All instincts warned me to stay away. Although she never looked sad, I knew she must have been hurting deep down. She was young, ten years younger than me. She had time to meet someone. I wasn't sure she'd notice me in any romantic sense.

"I clocked Charlie straight away." Said Helen. "Ha, how could you not notice those beautiful but sad eyes? Right away, I felt this overwhelming urge to make her smile. I wanted those eyes to smile too."

Meanwhile, I thought she seemed young, maybe too young. She said she liked my eyes. I felt the first stirrings of attraction. It had been so long. Breathe, Charlie, just breathe.

"Perhaps I came across as silly and flighty; she didn't seem too keen at first. I did manage to make her laugh, though," recalled Helen.

Helen was a breath of fresh air, so cheerful and fun. I looked forward to the end of the day when she'd pop into the office to say hi to everyone. I wanted to get to know her, but I was all too aware of our differences. She'd been married before...to a man.

"Charlie looked good for her age; lean, wiry, a typical runner's build. No sense of style though; her outfits needed a bit of colour."

Helen usually wore track bottoms and polo shirts, the usual garb of sports teachers. However, it didn't hide the fact that her body looked good; curvy but athletic. A skilled hockey player too, I'd watched her on the pitch.

"A slow burn is what we were. I flirted outrageously. I thought I'd made my interest in Charlie very clear at a staff get-together one evening. My outfit seemed to be the only thing that sparked her attention. Bright colours to match my happy mood!"

Helen looked incredible at our staff social. I told her so. She joked that I could do with a bit more colour in my life. I agreed, assuming she meant my choice of clothing. Talk turned to relationships. Leaning in like co-conspirators as we debated the merits of monogamy versus singledom. She explained that her ex had moved to the city for work. "Good riddance and all that" is how she felt about it. With no immediate family on his side, this felt like the end of a chapter for her. Happy to be in her presence, I listened but shared little of my experiences. That evening, I confided in Duke the attraction I felt towards her. He turned his mournful eyes to me and seemed to agree.

I was still running, just not very often. I hadn't done a race in a while, so I thought, why not? I started bringing my running kit to school. I'd run from there. The joys of living in the countryside mean trails for miles. On one of these occasions, Helen asked if she could join me.

"If, at first, you don't succeed, try and try...running! My repertoire of jokes and funny stories made her laugh, but that's where it ended. She was going to make me do all the work. After all the flirty banter, we agree to run together."

She wants to join me on a trail run. I warn her that it requires a different fitness level and ability. We laugh when I say I'll go easy on her.

"I'm fit and fast; ask anyone on the hockey team, but my goodness, I struggled to keep up. After four miles at a brisk pace, I was puffing," Helen revealed.

What was Helen thinking? After a few miles, she glowed... bright red, like a tomato. At first, she claimed she had a stitch; later, she needed to stretch. As she stood there looking rather hot and flustered, I knew then that I would do anything to be with her. Cautiously, I asked her out then, and she agreed. Rather enthusiastically, to my relief.

We haven't looked back since.

It took only a few weeks of dating before we both agreed that we felt a strong connection. So Helen moved in with me. At our age, we knew what we wanted, so why wait? Skip ahead five years, and here we are. Still laughing, still running, and deeply in love.

We now live in a beautifully restored period cottage just outside town. Duke, my ageing rescue, has joined Doris, another rescue. She is a bundle of joy, bringing high jinks and laughter into our lives. Helen chose her. They make quite a pair, in stark contrast to the thoughtful, serious duo that is Duke and me. Helen is also responsible for turning this formerly dark and dank cottage into a bright and cheerful home that is mainly tidy and usually clean. Her hockey kit sometimes clutters the hallways, and our washing machine forever hums its familiar tunes in the background. Our Friday curry nights with friends and Helen's hockey club socials at the weekend are a part of our weekly routine. Overall, the life I've wanted for a long, long time.

So why the hesitation, you ask? Well, my age is creeping up on me. My achy joints are a constant reminder that I am the older one. It has me questioning whether I should be retiring the distance running. Helen, years younger, rather annoyingly, passes me by easily now and shouts, "Keep up, old lady". I'd usually bounce back relatively quickly after a lengthy run, but I'm noticing it's no longer easy. Even with all the energy supplements, running has become hard work.

Oh, and this only recently. She wants a baby. It's what she's wanted for a long time. We'd spoken about it over the years. She admits this is one of the reasons her marriage failed. She could not trust him as a husband, even less as a father. It's the main reason we adopted Doris. A way to satisfy Helen's nurturing side. She thinks that having a baby will deepen our relationship. Not that I doubt her commitment to me. She knows that I have been hurt in the past. If I'm being honest, I initially worried that she was in a hetero relationship before. It made me question her motives at first. Now I trust her with all my heart. I've even proposed marriage to her *twice*. She will not marry again. She's made that abundantly clear. "Once bitten, twice shy. Besides, been there done that," is all she'll say about that.

I'm just not sure what a baby will mean for us. It feels like the ultimate commitment. There's no going back from that. But can this mean Helen sees me as her forever after? Dare I believe that she is mine forever? I want so desperately to believe this.

Let's assume we go ahead as per her plan. I haven't had a period in over a year, so I know *I'm* menopausal. Naturally, Helen offered to bear the child using a sperm donor. That makes sense. Is my hesitation going to jeopardise what we have? Another concern is we will soon have to part with Duke. While he has shown no signs of slowing down, he is an old guy, and his achy joints reflect that. It feels like a lot to take in right now. These are significant decisions.

"Charlie, time is of the essence, and my clock is ticking. Loudly!" insists Helen. "Stop overthinking it!"

She's got a point. Already life has changed as we knew it, post-pandemic.

"All the more reason to plan for the future," says Helen.

But how do I let go of my past so that it doesn't spoil my future?

I suppose my fear and reluctance also stem from the 'blast from the past' telephone call I received near the end of the lockdown. We'd been coping well with everything Covid related. The enforced lockdown was bearable, and although I liked working from home, I also missed the staff room chats. The dogs, however, loved their new routine and soon found themselves under my desk by day. Helen used this time to declutter and organise the store cupboards. No cupboard went unnoticed and untouched. She also did all the food shops, not just for us, but for our ageing parents and our elderly neighbours as well. Mother looked forward to the end of the week when Helen would pop by with her groceries and have a natter from the end of the garden. "Such a kind girl, our Helen. Charlie hit the jackpot with her."

I knew she was careful as she wore her mask and kept her distance, but not having any physical contact with them was hard. She's such a tactile person. The dogs and I gave her loads of kisses and cuddles. Being a sports teacher meant she was initially furloughed. This gave Helen much-needed time to read, mainly cookbooks, and soon she was baking and experimenting with ingredients that suddenly seemed in high demand.

And then, one day, an unknown number called on my phone. I took it.

"Is that you, Charlotte? Darling, how are you? Where've you been all my life? I've missed you."

Helen had been working in the kitchen but had heard the French-accented voice as I'd turned up the volume and speaker on my phone. She appeared at my side in an instant. I've shared every detail of my past with her. She knew immediately who this was.

"Darling, I must see you one last time. I want to look into those soulful dark eyes of yours again."

"The only way you're going to see her is at the end of a video call, if only to tell her to fuck off!" muttered Helen angrily.

"Switch on your camera, ma Cherie," Cara insisted.

I'm not sure what I'm expecting to see. The Cara of my youth? The Cara that still captivates, full of the same insatiable energy? No, that's not possible. I hesitate, but I turn the camera on. Instead, I see an older woman. **A shrivelled-up husk of an older woman.** A caricature of her former self. Age and a life of excess had not been kind to her. But, even if this was the old Cara, I am no longer the old Charlie. The way forward is brighter.

"Rusty old banger isn't she?" says Helen off camera and out of earshot. She's right. Gone are the sleek lines of the Jaguar, this ravager of my youth. It's she who's been ravaged. Her hedonism has finally caught up with her. She is dying of cancer.

At first, I'm repulsed by her.

Then I pity her.

Finally, I forgive her.

| 7 |

Ageing and Ageism: Interviews in the West, East, and somewhere in between

The West...

What does ageing mean for women in your country?

Past: I can only speak from what I know. My mamma was born in 1936 in Buckhannon, a pretty coalmining town to the Northeast of West Virginia. My daddy was a coal miner and raised to be a man's man. Both my parents were proud of State and country. We've always been church-going Methodists. My folks married young, and with four kids, my mamma was happy to be at home. She got involved in the community and loved it. In our small town, everyone knows everyone. We're super friendly around here, with non-stop swapping stories while chewing the cud at the gatherings. We're proud to call ourselves rednecks.

My daddy died in a car accident before his cancer got him. My mamma died of a heart attack in her early seventies. It was no surprise, our love of sugar and hard labouring. Many of her friends have died the same way- too soon and as poor widows. My parents had seen many changes in our district. We've gone from a booming coal mining town with a guaranteed paycheck to more of us on the breadline. We're not a ghost town yet; our coalmines are still open. Some folks say there is probably another ten years' worth in the seams. Of course, when you call yourself a coalminer, they say you're a polluter. Anyhow, we don't believe in global warming.

Present: I knew that I wanted more things than my mamma. I married young and had my kids early. Once my girls went to school, I joined my husband in running our diner. Everything was going nicely, and then Covid hit, and it hit hard around here. That's how I lost my husband. Now I run it with my oldest daughter. I love my community. I know everyone who eats my food. Everyone loves it, but I'm watching all of us getting fatter, even after the warnings following Covid. It isn't funny now that I've been diagnosed with diabetes. I guess I'm guilty of serving the food that is slowly killing us all. Not anymore. I've recently been on our local news with my 'fresh is best' and plant-based menu—the first of its kind. I'm on my feet all day but not especially active. I try and look after myself more than my mamma did. I take an exercise class every week and return to the slimming club when the slaw dogs and pepperoni rolls jump into my mouth. I worry about my friends. We've all got some health complaints, and the healthcare system is bad. That's why most of us have taken out health insurance. The pandemic was a wake-up call for all. Folks out in the sticks were cut off as the WIFI was non-existent. Even when you get a signal, it's slow and expensive. Maybe that's why our young folk are leaving the state—that, and the poverty, drugs, and the high suicide rate. Not me; I was born here, and I'll die here.

Future: My oldest daughter is a maxi me; her waist is even bigger than mine. She will take over the diner when I retire, eventually. Like me, she's tied to this place. My youngest is already more educated than I am. She graduated from West Virginia University and now works in Pittsburgh; so close but so far apart. Her world is so different from her sister's.

For a start, she's a vegetarian. Guess who is a fan of the healthy menu in the diner? No matter; I'm proud of her. She's blazing a trail. I'm also proud of my oldest. She understands around these parts; it's all about the small wins. I'm gonna be a grandmamma soon. My girls barely remember their grandma, so I want to be around for the next generation. We've got the community; we need to fight for better understanding. Change is slow.

Does ageism exist? How do the young perceive the old?

Once you hit your forties around here, you are on the downward slope and collecting speed. If you're lucky to live a long life, you're a long time old, and you'll be on medication. If you're a female, it's a scary place to be. Most of us live and die alone. If you're disabled and can't move, it makes you needy and miserable.

So if I'm honest, our young see getting old as getting slow, sick, ignored, and unhappy. We're shamed for not taking better care of ourselves. Besides, they feel like they'll pick up the tab—a hefty tab. I think the whole country is chasing youth. Why? If you're young, you can participate at every level in society, you're independent, you're not marginalised, and more importantly, you don't share their space. Chasing youth around here is always going to be a losing battle.

Is your country facing a 'Silver Tsunami?'

Well, I guess so now that you've explained what that means. West Virginia is greying, and our young are leaving. But we still have a high teenage pregnancy rate around here, and we're anti-abortion.

I know of the health and social care crisis, so my family is covered by private health. And the national pension pot is running low. I hear about that all the time, but I think I'm gonna be all right.

If so, what is your country/state doing to mitigate the crisis?

Honestly, I'm not sure what the rest of the state is doing. There are huge public awareness campaigns out there. In these parts, there are hot meal deliveries to older folk and transportation to medical appointments. I've had to put up the new nutritional guidelines in our diner. So there's a lot of information out there about staying healthy. But it's hard.

On the one hand, they're telling us what we should be doing, but on the other, they're still making doorways and access ramps wider. Ain't nobody here wants to change or give up our local treats anytime soon. Let's just say the healthy options on the diner menu are not building my pension pot.

How is all this filtering down to you?

Here and there, I'm seeing messages about living better for longer. Some of these messages are helpful, and some are downright scary. Unfortunately, I only listened when I got my diagnosis. Don't get me wrong, most of us are too busy living our lives to notice any symptoms creeping in. It will take a lot more than billboard messages because old habits die hard. Besides, it's a weighty issue.

Podcaster: Pun unintended, thank you.

The East... (as translated)

What does ageing mean for women in your country?

Past: My mother was born before WWII (1940) and was raised in a rural matriarchal household. But this ended with the premature deaths of her parents. As a teenager, she was sent to live with family in Osaka. Here, societal expectations were that she should marry and have children. In Japanese society, it is an important step toward becoming an adult. That's how she met my father a few years later. It was an arranged marriage. He was educated. Following the war years, America strongly influenced Japanese culture. He was a traditionalist, expecting her to remain home and raise their offspring. I was an only child. Women like my mother have a high status in our society. Her role as wife allowed her to make household decisions and control the household budget. She could vote and even divorce and remarry if she wished. She didn't; she remained true. Legally, she was equal to my father; however, culturally, she was required to submit. First to her father (had he lived), secondly, to her husband (and she did), and thirdly to any sons borne into this marriage. Although this seems restrictive, by virtue of her age and status, she was and remains valued by all.

My parents live close by. Our families live on the first floor of the same city apartment block. A stroke of fortune meant that an apartment two doors away became available just as my parents began to need more help. My father was becoming frail and needed constant nursing care. He suffers from heart disease and has been hospitalised for a while now. We worry that he will soon leave us. The men in his family have all died from heart attacks. My mother recently had a fall, and they discovered that she has osteoporosis. Now I worry all the time about her falling down the stairs. My husband's parents have always lived with us. Although both grannies require assistance, they have AI-assisted mechanical aids in the home. They remain largely independent. Relying on each other to navigate public transport, they remain active in our community. My mother-in-law occasionally helps me cook and still insists on visiting the markets daily for fresh ingredients. Our lives are more enriched by having our parents close. We feel duty-bound to care for them financially, and we do so selflessly. Fortunately, they will provide us with an inheritance to allow for this not to impact our financial situation.

Present: I feel privileged that my parents encouraged me to study and could pay for my studies. I have a teaching degree. Yet, I have always been conflicted. My mother felt I should have stayed home after having my daughter; to be a dutiful wife and mother. I wanted that but I also wanted to continue adding value to society. Teaching felt like my destiny. My daughter grew up with me working daily and doing the evening household chores. Even with my in-laws' help, I cared for her when she was young. Childcare was expensive and was needed for me to work, and somehow we managed. Now she is at a university in Tokyo. I still do most of the household chores and take care of the budget. Plus, I continued to look after both sets of parents, which can be exhausting, so I retired early. I remain in good health. I accept that my role is to continue creating a harmonious family life. My husband has an important job in the bank. He works long hours. He is always feeling stressed out and fatigued. Our lifestyle may continue in this way for a little longer. There is talk that the retirement age will be extended to seventy years. I don't think he minds this. It will keep him busy.

Future: My daughter is pursuing her master's degree in social sciences. She has very modern ideas. Her reluctance to marry young comes from her knowledge of the responsibilities that I have always had. There is no stigma associated with being single amongst her generation as it was with mine. She also feels that gender equality is lacking in the corporate world. It is where she sees her future. She constantly reminds me that more women like her must be business leaders. Young female business leaders are a minority group at the moment. Her ideal partner is one who, in addition to being supportive of her career, will share the responsibilities of house and childcare. Perhaps even be the stay-at-home dad. I hope that she finds that particular person soon. The men she's been meeting seem intimidated by her. I feel confident that her intentions to be a modern career woman will not clash with her respect for the traditional ways. Her future may look a little different.

Does ageism exist? How do the young perceive the old?

I would say, on the whole, there are no prejudices against our older generation. We have an elevated level of social cohesion. However, our young people are worried they may have to shoulder the financial burden of healthcare. Japan's fertility rates are falling, and our replacement generational gap is widening. This growing concern of a skills shortage will need to be bridged somehow. Our government has plans to ensure that older people remain valued in employment and society. There are many centres for social care, and some are very modern. For now, I have my checklist and follow all the health initiatives for women my age. When my daughter comes home in the holidays, she joins her grandmothers at the local park where they practice Tai Chi, along with many other elderly residents. The younger generation has a lot of respect for their elders. It is how it has always been and how it will continue to be.

Is your country facing a 'Silver Tsunami?'

If you mean, are there more older people than young people in our country, then yes. But I can only speak for my community. Where we live, it does feel like there are more people my age (50+) and older around. We mainly see our young people in the inner-city areas. Our rural areas are becoming extinct. So yes, overall, we are facing an ever-widening generation gap.

Podcaster: Japan currently has the world's fastest ageing society (65+) with the largest super-aged demographic (70+).

If so, what is your country/state doing to mitigate the crisis?

There are many government initiatives in place. This is what I've found out from the following two sources:

(Towards a third term of Health Japan 21 and The Lancet Regional Health – Western Pacific.)

An initiative called 'Healthy Japan 21' was launched in 2013. It is a ten-year plan with the following goals:

- To extend healthy life expectancy
- To reduce health disparities across local governments
- To have accountability tables for all
- To reduce Japan's healthcare expenditure

Another initiative called 'Community-based integrated care system' was launched in 2012. These stakeholder levels are involved:

- Individuals and families – known as Self-help (Ji Jo)
- Community volunteers – known as Mutual aid (Go Jo)

- Organised social and security programmes – known as Social solidarity care (Kyo Jo)
- Public medical and welfare systems and public assistance funded by tax revenues – known as Governmental care (Ko Jo)

The overall goals for Japan's future focus on the following:

- Healthy active individuals
- Community-based integrated Care by 2025
- Municipal autonomy
- All of the above will contribute to Japan becoming the global health leader—the health model for other countries by 2035

How is all this filtering down to you?

Podcaster: I understand that Japan is one of the most advanced countries in the world regarding digital connectivity, social media usage, and mobile connectivity. How does this work for you and your family?

Well, some of our homes have robots many care homes have them too. So we have welcomed this addition to our labour force. Firstly we do not fear them. Secondly, we trust that the development and safety protocols are strictly evaluated when this technology reaches the end user. So I do not have any concerns with AI assistance, should I need it.

Podcaster: AI is coming whether we want it or not. However, it will never replace the human touch.

Somewhere In Between...

What does ageing mean for women in your country?

Past: My mother was born in the war years 1937. She grew up with rationing and fear. Her narrative is that she was brought up with humble expectations. She still considers herself a traditionalist more than a moderniser and is very pragmatic.

She adored her father, who was kind but patriarchal. He had different expectations for daughters and sons. Her mother was modest and a capable homemaker. But, on reflection, she was an uncelebrated drudge.

My mother has a keen sense of family and values; her dream/ expectation was to fall in with the norms of the time: to be a good housewife and mother.

Church provided the moral backdrop and a sense of community, along with the tennis club and lawn bowls. She valued decent food on the table, cleanliness to keep disease at bay, and grooming to demonstrate self-care and self-respect.

My father's affairs meant divorce and enormous stress for her. A single mother in the 1960s had a stigma attached. She suddenly had to find employment but discovered she was more capable than she thought. Having proved herself to be resilient, she then became fiercely independent. Her routines and various rituals maintain her sense of self and well-being. Even now, she continues to do so. She lives alone but makes considerable efforts to actively contribute to her family and her village. She's one of the lucky ones because others are falling thick and fast around her. There is a palpable and abject fear of going into a home. She has recently seen two of her female friends end up in a care home with dementia. She worries about losing her autonomy and being diminished. It would feel like the end of the line. As her siblings and friends succumb to old age and pass, she's now witnessing her community shrink. Still, she continues to live well and is determined to enjoy life and its possibilities.

Present: My legacy from my mother's generation is gratitude and an appreciation of the opportunities for women like me. I live in a democracy with the legal right to vote and the right to be fully educated. In addition, I am entitled to equal pay and access to birth control and to be the mistress of my body. In other words, my future has lots of possibilities with fewer restrictions than my mother's generation. Yet, middle age brings its challenges.

I still feel vital and sexy. I know that I need to look after my health, physical and mental. I'm bombarded with what to do and how to do it, and still, I don't always get it right. Recently it felt like life is assaulting me. I've lost a friend to cancer, endured many bad dates in my quest to find another life partner, and had a personal health scare. I'm striking a balance between a nurturing parent and a libertarian one. My wish is to enable my young to fledge without burden whilst I remain strong and not too needy. My mission is to continue role-modelling what ageing well looks like.

My professional network allows me to keep my finger on the pulse. I feel encouraged by the advances in nutrition and medicine, but both are not going fast enough for me. Thank God for our Healthcare System, a safety net for all.

As a member of the sandwich generation, I take my responsibility seriously. I am a conduit for both the past and the future generations. For now, in my own family, I aim to bridge this ever-increasing gap.

As a journalist and podcaster, I intend to spread the word.

Future: My children are future-focused and less interested in learning from the past. They have moments of curiosity, and certainly, their playlists indicate that they still admire my generation's pop culture. Yet, when it comes to their health, what I'm seeing is at odds with what they're feeling. In this period of constant mental and physical flux, somewhere in the shadows lurks potential danger. What will healthy ageing look like for them in the future? I can only guess.

Will it depend on their socio-economic profile? Will their various apps drive it? Or is it more guided by their connectivity? This sense of connection is both in real life and in the digital world—a dual existence: the tangible and the virtual.

But what do young people say? First, they'll explain digital connectivity. To them, it's simply an encompassing term for mobile and fixed Internet connections. 'Hardware', in our day, but let's get it right, 'devices' in theirs. But what does it represent? EVERY-THING!

In 2012 creeping into BOOM came social media. Now playing across all devices. For all generations. Can we imagine a time without it?

Let's explore this with my journalistic fall back - Kipling's 'six honest serving ...Women.'

What – are the platforms?

Instagram, Facebook, Twitter, Snapchat, TikTok, Be Real, and many more.

Why use these?

Schools encourage fact-finding, problem-solving,

It gives our young social connection, provides entertainment, and allows creativity.

From a mature stance, it's more of a functional tool, but for our young, it's a much bigger deal. A digital presence helps to create a personal brand that contributes to their sense of self.

When are they using it?

Pretty much all the time, that device is another limb, and let's face it, aren't we all a bit addicted? The searches alone are seductive. An occasional search has the potential to open the floodgate to needless information. The constant pings and alerts demonstrate a sense of urgency, and along with that comes a response protocol. When the inner circle of contacts and influencers beckons, and you miss an experience, opportunity, information, or a drop, heaven forbid you'd got it wrong. Take the speed of response to messages, for example. Too long and it's misinterpreted; too short and it means you're needy. Let's not even talk about those blue ticks with no comeback. These new bedtime companions give us our last closing thought and our first waking moment.

How does it make them feel?

They feel accepted and understood. Always on it, always ready. They are connected with no fear of missing out (FOMO), submerging in this maelstrom of data superfluous or otherwise, weary and overwhelmed; our instinct is to throw them a lifeline. Extricate only, not exit.

Where? Anywhere where there is a connection. See the rise of the digital nomads.

Who is using it? Anyone with a device.

Now the loaded **Why.** Why is this a problem for our young?

Firstly without us knowing enough, they are left to their own devices. Literally. In the early days, 11-13 years, schools will have a series of safeguarding sessions, '*How to keep your child safe.*' But then, before you realise it, they're off. Launched into a digital arena and guided by their friends, who are also in free fall. All learning from their own mistakes. Are they sharing too freely without payback, checks, or balances? Are their naïve honesties and candid discussions protected, or are they facing a toxic backlash in isolation? Selfies that lead to sexting and beyond. The pressure to conform is immense in the hook-up culture created by social media. Revenge porn is a consequence of trust gone wrong. Viral posts happen all the time. Social norms present in face-to-face exchanges seem to vanish in the virtual world. Are they aware of the power they place in unsafe hands? Labels can damage and are hard to shrug off. I'm sure my lot has shielded me from what goes on in their digital lives. They recognise that my knee-jerk reaction could result in a moral panic, judging without fully understanding the nature of the menace. So while our young continue to focus on the positives, and there are many, we as parents are increasingly tuning in to the negatives:

- sleep deprivation
- low mood
- social comparisons
- body image issues (self-objectification)
- eating disorders
- low self-esteem

But much more so than the usual teen angst. Because coupled with fewer 'in-person social interactions' across generations, the hidden toll on their health is often overlooked. No wonder granny curses their preoccupation with their devices rather than being present in the moment.

So how did we get here?

High-income English-speaking countries value independence and innovation, but are we guilty of taking our eye off the ball and leaving our younger generation to it? Maybe. Study after study in these countries confirms that the growing mental health crisis crashes between the ages of 14 and 17, especially for girls. It's even got its term, SMD= social media disorder. The sedentary nature of digital connectivity isn't helping our obesity crisis either. Through these platforms, they are also flooded by other anxiety-provoking world events:

- climate change
- natural disasters
- pandemics
- economic recession
- healthcare crisis
- human right issues
- and wars

In this space, in real-time, viral posts can potentially lead to negative contagion. At this hormonal age, moods are variable and easily triggered by events and stressors. Perspective is always the challenge. Am I naively trusting the regulators to police this growing menace outside of the safety of the home? Surely I'm not alone in my concern. Social media is evolving and is here to stay. We need to master it rather than allow it to master us. Who puts the damn genie back in the bottle?

Despite my efforts, I still get the occasional "Your generation wouldn't understand," so I ask, "Why wouldn't we?" and then try to do so. After all, the more I am interested, the more they're likely to share their interests. And, with that recognition, I enable my mother to stay digitally connected too. After all, no one should be left behind.

And to finally answer the question, 'What does healthy ageing mean for the future?' Well, it comes down to choices. So exactly like you would operate an app: Connect or disconnect. Enable or disable. Give and take. Navigate. Extricate.

Does ageism exist? How do the young perceive the old?

I'm not aware of it in my own family. We haven't written Granny off yet. We wouldn't dare to. From a more comprehensive view, age discrimination is not just unfair but illegal in this country. And yet, it's everywhere; it represents the most significant discrimination here. The negative portrayal of older people has strongly influenced societal perceptions. They are denigrated and seen as frail and in decline. Think about the advertising posters on public transport and television using older people to sell funeral plans. Or doubting their competence by using more senior people in targeted awareness campaigns involving scams. These negative attitudes and perceptions exist across all levels of society, sometimes hidden, often blatantly obvious. There is a risk that this narrative will continue to colour the judgement of our young.

With higher age numbers synonymous with being fragile, vulnerable, and dependent, in other words, a cost, it's no wonder ageism exists.

It's time to *reframe* what ageing should look and feel like. Reframing means it should be about ageing healthily and living a life of purpose. Rather than defying age, we, as a society, should accept it and adapt accordingly. It then becomes less about cultural, financial, and social burdens and more about the lasting value and continued participation across all generations.

Is your country facing a 'Silver Tsunami?'

From my research, YES. First, let's start by changing that metaphor. Tsunami sounds catastrophic and invokes age-panic and fear. So let's not panic. Let's get real instead. Think RIPPLES rather than crashing waves. It is better to view this ageing demographic with a broader conceptual shift. Ideally, ripples of positive interventions flow across all levels of society, reaching different individuals at various times. Government and policymakers create structures that enable individuals to thrive, adapting to find their level of happiness. Always recognising that each person will have their context, be it gender, race, sexuality, class, or wealth. Not forgetting each has distinct levels of agency too.

But ageing and ageing well are complex constructs. For too long, the onus has been on the deserving individual to shoulder moral responsibility by adopting correct behaviours and attitudes that determine active ageing to good health. Unfortunately, we're not all able to do so.

We should no longer view healthy ageing as a business model with profit and productivity as the primary focus. The dilemma is being human.

Instead, let's capture the essence of the older individual. Let's be **age positive**. Reconfiguring their value in terms of knowledge, experience, and wisdom. While taking an active role in the ageing process is down to us, it requires an operational infrastructure to support us. With all of this in mind, our measures of success as individuals and societies can be chartered on the happiness scale. Japan has done this already. And so has Finland and Denmark. It is possible.

If so, what is your country/state doing to mitigate the crisis?

Globally, we've already started the World Health Organisation's (WHO) Decade of Healthy Ageing. How many of us even knew about the campaign, never mind that we are already two years into it? What is it all about?

Governments, educators, and industries worldwide are responsible for interpreting the noble aims of this campaign. Our challenge in this country is considering what that means for our multicultural population. We accept that the roll-out plan is complex. We will know that the efforts of the stakeholders and the champions responsible for implementing this crusade are on target when it's common parlance when the information trickles down to us. And when the outcomes are less talked about but more felt. In other words, it finds us rather than we reach for it. What are the benchmarks?

At the moment, it's down to us to join the dots. We need a real-time barometer in one space. We all need to pay attention. Already there is a growing rhetoric about the dangers of poor health linked to the isolation of older people. We know that the retirement age has been extended. Now there is a call for earlier retirees to return to the workforce, albeit part-time. And at local levels, let's not leave anyone behind. We've covered the world, country, region, and local communities, and finally, let's address you and your bubble. This is what the average person needs to know about ageing.

Firstly, ignore the scaremongers. Fear doesn't help. Secondly, change your tone. The youth are new, the middle-aged are mature, the young old are vintage, and the senior old are simply priceless. Every age has its value, which grows, not diminishes. And thirdly, let's be kinder and more inclusive with our media campaigns. Not all of us are white, middle-class, educated, and funded. There are shades of wealth and shades of health in the ageing demographic too.

So to answer that question, are we doing enough to mitigate? In my opinion, not enough. As a nation, we have excellent charities that represent our ageing population.

Let's turn up the noise. To deafening volumes. Sorry Granny.

How is all this filtering down to you?

So what are the layers that affect me? In my circle, women my age and older balance their lives, pacing themselves. Some are ready to retire, and some cannot afford to. A few are using this stage of their lives to redefine their time and purpose, making constant adjustments and always being discerning about the value of their time.

How does that affect me? Now more than before, I witnessed how my industry and society generally deal with age. I want to be part of this movement for change, where anything is possible. We see octogenarians running marathons all the time. I must be an outlier too. Some of my friends involve themselves in charitable and local events. I do, too, when I can, but I want more. What's clear is we all still have a sense of purpose and a need to contribute. That's how my digital media broadcasting began. I went from a bustling news desk in the city to having quiet conversations in my homemade studio. Why? After many incidental everyday chats, and on the back of a suggestion: 'I wish I knew,' I had an epiphany. I needed to satisfy a growing need to understand and manage all aspects of ageing, women's health, and well-being. I've worked out that it starts with connectivity.

By luck or judgement, I've somehow achieved six levels of connection. Of course, my connectivity could have shrunk quickly with changes in age and circumstances. But I've actively built it up, including the digital kind.

Like many women, I've been thrown curveballs with unexpected life events and the expected. I've worked hard on controlling my stress and how I respond to adverse events emotionally. How much I absorb and how much I release. It's always going to be an effort. But I also finally get it; daily movement clears the head and strengthens the heart. It's not an option.

Health matters, so let's stay healthy.

Please tune in to our next media segment, this time a webinar. It's all about managing risk and why chasing the simple rewards matter.

| 8 |

Bella's story

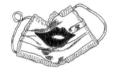

The low hum of machines and the snicking sound of Crocs on a polished linoleum floor shook me out of my dreamlike state. Back to work again, back to visiting those patients needing to be treated, wanting to be comforted, fearful of dying. The A&E alarm sounded its too-familiar warning, and the madness began again.

Triage, diagnose, intubate, and monitor.

I looked up and saw her. She was the fourth one in that morning. One of my people. She was in cardiac arrest and surrounded by emergency staff. I sensed the urgency; I felt their concern. They cared, and it showed. I know some of these colleagues well. We'd been fighting this battle for some time but covered in all the protective clothing and equipment; they seemed otherworldly, almost alien. Later, when they removed their visors and goggles, the compression marks left their faces swollen and bruised. I saw the fear and despair in their eyes. I knew mine reflected the same.

A few frantic moments passed, and they pronounced her—another Covid related death.

As I passed by her, I paused to look at her. She looked about fifty. She was voluptuous. She was still wearing her street clothes. I straightened her braids and tucked her skirt under her legs, restoring her dignity. Who are you? Do your loved ones know that you're here? I wondered.

It suddenly dawned on me; this could be me.

No time to think. The alarm sounded again, and we were off once more.

Triage, diagnose, intubate, and monitor.

Later that day, in a lull, *when it felt like we could breathe again,* one of the nurses used lipstick to draw a big red smile on the outside of her mask. Soon, we were all doing it, doctors and consultants alike. It cheered us up to no end. Those were the light-hearted moments that kept us going. They were the rays of sunshine in a room filled with darkness. Some of our less critically ill patients felt our good cheer, and they gave us a thumbs up.

A shift change after another harrowing day, fourteen hours long. We decamped to the changing station, where we shrugged off our anxiety, our exhaustion, and our protective clothing. The weariness in the locker room was palpable. We struggled to find those tiny sparks of hope and strength to carry to our families on the outside. Masks went on again. That we were even going home, felt like an achievement. Patients, colleagues and friends had been lost along the way.

In the car park, as we prepared to leave, we stopped and observed the social distance while taking a moment to share a silent prayer for the endless stream of ambulances arriving at the entrance to the A&E. Stretcher after stretcher was being unloaded as members of the public were taken through the doors to the Covid wards. The struggle continued. I cracked open the car window and, for a second, enjoyed the fresh air. My face felt puffy, my skin dry and itchy, and my eyes gritty. I'm relieved to be going home. I thought, *...in You we trust,* as I drove away. *No time to process, to question decisions. Too tired, must recharge.* Tomorrow I will be back again. Hearing. Seeing. Smelling. Stress, distress, here on the frontline, as we fought.

Christian, my husband, waited at the window for me. We touched and kissed through the glass. I saw the concern in his eyes. He saw fear in mine. It had been this way since the start of the pandemic when we first realised how infectious this virus was. He assured me that our son was well and asleep, and he had once again asked if I was coming home. I longed to wrap my arms around them but knew this was impossible. Not yet, not until we were out of the woods. He blew me a kiss. Reluctantly I turned away and went to the granny flat where Mum had been living until recently. We were one of the lucky ones if you can call it that. Some of my colleagues were sleeping in tents in their gardens. Mum moved back into the house to look after my family. I occupied her space now. I carried the burden of risk every time I left the hospital. So far, so good. They've left my dinner in a container by the door. Usually, there is a note attached to it from Christian, and a drawing, always a multi-coloured rainbow, from my boy. This time, I found an envelope with 'thank you cards' from everyone on my street. Each one is covered with a protective plastic sleeve. These gestures so touched me that I burst into tears. It all poured out, the sadness, the worry, the exhaustion. Later, as I drifted to sleep, I once again prayed, *do not forsake us.*

This multi-ethnic neighbourhood in Birmingham is where I have grown up and now live. I've come full circle, first leaving to study and later returning with a husband and a profession. These people, my people, share the same values, love the same foods, and experience the same discriminations and prejudices. My parents were Jamaican immigrants. Leroy and Mary. They were part of the Windrush generation arriving in the UK in the early sixties and met after moving to the north of England. Dad worked in construction, and Mum worked for the NHS, first as a health worker, then later as a nurse. A few years after I was born, Dad tragically died when scaffolding collapsed on a building site. I was too young to remember anything from that time, but Mum ensured he stayed alive in our thoughts and memories.

Your Dad was a good man, Bella; he took such loving care of us. After you were born, he would tell everyone at work that he was going home to his beautiful ladies. Unlike some of the other husbands, if he wasn't working, he didn't mind looking after you. It allowed me to finish my studies. He was so proud of me when I graduated. A modern man he was. He had such big plans. "Mary," he'd say, "I'm going to build you the house of your dreams, like the one your mum used to live in back home. I will grow palm trees here, and you can have your vegetable garden. Anything for you, my queen, Mary."

Although I was too young to remember him, through Mum's words, I continue to feel a deep connection with him. His spirit remains ever present in my life.

How he liked to tease me, Bella. "This country is so cold, Mary; I have never worn so many clothes. What happens when I want to hug you? How will you feel, my love?" Then he would grab my hand and place it over his manly bump.

Hearing my mother say these words, I sensed their love for each other. Yet, I also understood from her sometimes-sad eyes how upsetting it must have been to have lost him so early on.

My formative years were colourful. The council estate we lived on was a poor substitute for the Caribbean landscape that many residents had left behind. Still, it was rich with the culture and the ever-positive spirit of these first- and second-generation citizens. As a hardworking, single mother, Mum relied heavily on her friends. Only a few family members had come over with her from Jamaica. All, including the aunties, shared the responsibility of raising me. They nourished and nurtured simultaneously. My soft, dimpled little body was a testament to the delicious, lovingly cooked meals that made their way to our table. As I grew older in this protective bubble, I was shielded from the injustices of the time. Mum made sure of that. She had first-hand experience of the ugliness and cruelty of ignorant people, even in the hospital where she worked. Dirty looks and hurtful remarks were plentiful, and yet Mum persevered.

Why did they invite us here if they didn't want to be treated by us?

Like any protective mother, she created a safe environment for me and fiercely controlled any content I was exposed to, sometimes even restricting television access. But, unfortunately, it still didn't stop me from hearing racist chants on the streets.

"Go back to your own country" and "Black people are taking our jobs" were just a few slurs spewed out by pale, angry faces.

In this mainly self-contained neighbourhood, we had each other's backs, so young and naïve, I believed that the rest of society did too. Only in junior school did I have my first real exposure to the harsh realities. I was afforded those first interactions between different ethnicities in school, which weren't always positive. As children, our elders had taught us not to draw attention to ourselves, that being stared at and whispered about spoke of the newness of our people to this country. I became used to questions about the colour of my skin and the texture of my hair. Even so, the school was exciting. As an only child, I welcomed my peers' company and lapped up our lessons' content. Those early years were happy ones, leaving no adverse memories.

As I entered my teens, the reality of life as a Black person became clear—too many stories of abuse and discrimination. I had considered myself fortunate thus far. But, unfortunately, this wasn't the case for the many young Black men in our midst. When the riots of Brixton happened in the early eighties, it set off a chain of events in our community. Suddenly, many more incidents spoke of the racial tightrope they were walking. These injustices and the hostile climate it created coincided with the start of my secondary schooling. For me, this time of growth, education and opportunity was also a time of loss, damage and destruction for many. Nevertheless, it marked the start of a new era. This newfound awareness of how the world was, and its treatment of people of colour, made me wary and sceptical for a while.

By nature, though, I am curious and willing to learn. Towards the end of my schooling, this optimistic and cheerful person I had grown into had had a relationship with a Black guy and then a White guy. Apart from the physical differences, I was left feeling liked, loved even, but equally betrayed by both. My heart and spirit remained intact, though; I played the long game regarding matters of the heart and life.

Mum had a pivotal role back then. By day she worked as a nurse in the local hospital, and twice a week, she helped run the women's clinic at our local centre. She was also part of the Gospel choir in church on Sundays. Her faith which sat neatly alongside her education and experience, made her a valued and influential member of this community. One of the elders, to be heard and respected. Her desire to do good and to acknowledge each member meant that at times I had to share her with friends, neighbours and even strangers. Yet she always was available to listen to me and, when she couldn't help, made sure to find someone who could. These values she instilled in me then contributed to my becoming a doctor.

In the early days of her retirement, Mum kept herself busy baking celebration cakes for weddings, birthdays, and christenings. Her boozy rum and coconut cakes were in huge demand. Coming home to a slice of her spicy almond cake was always a special treat. Over the years, these treats have become healthier versions of their predecessors. She was diagnosed with Type 2 diabetes soon after retiring and having cared for people with diabetes in the hospital; she knew enough about their suffering to know that she didn't want it for herself. However, she was determined to live well beyond retirement and wanted to use her voice to help promote a healthier lifestyle for all. That is how she started her little business, first by baking sugar-free alternatives for the family and then soon after having to meet the ever-increasing orders of her friends and ex-colleagues. Early efforts were interesting as she experimented with what she called 'Western ingredients.'

Healthy choices healthy life is her favourite mantra. She carries these thoughts and ideas into her social gatherings. Often, I find myself at the receiving end of her disapproving looks and shaking her head as she points out my decidedly unhealthy choices. After Mum was given a clean bill of health, she turned her attention to me.

Bella, you know better. When are you going to take care of yourself?

Agreeing with her was an easy route to harmony. Yet it always prompted me to start an eating plan, and achieve somewhat moderate success, followed by disappointment that I'd let myself down. AGAIN. Over the years, it has become a pattern. Mum will notice that I'm faltering and will not always subtly remind me; my knee-jerk reaction is to join a slimming group or start a plan of my own. Which usually spurs me on for another month or two. After which, in a moment of weakness, I sabotage my efforts or, as described in the world of slimming, 'revert to type.'

My coping mechanism at times of stress is to comfort eat. I am also not averse to the guilty pleasure of a tipple or two. It's the perfect juxtaposition of being in control while simultaneously losing control. I know no other way.

In my junior doctor years, when time was a luxury, the way I thought about food changed. Instead of being savoured and enjoyed in a relaxed social context, it became a hurried and guilty individual pleasure. I always knew what I ought to eat, but my reality was a little different. My work schedule didn't permit me to follow predictable eating patterns, and the availability of healthy choices was a constant challenge. Grab-and-go meals in hospital canteens consisted of stodgy sandwiches, crisps and sugary drinks. My sweet tooth also meant I was supplementing an already dodgy diet with plenty of sweet treats. As for exercise, that just wasn't an option for me. No time. Besides, I considered being run off my feet all day, every day, a strenuous workout. My downtime was all about catching up on much-needed sleep.

Before the Covid pandemic, the medical profession was already dealing with the consequences of the obesity epidemic. News headlines linked the two, meaning we all contribute to the statistics. As healthcare staff, we saw first-hand the scale of the problem. Covid became a wake-up call for all of us for differing reasons. The fear and the forced isolation drove many to reach out, socialise, and indulge even more. We were all bombarded on social media with our collective baking and cooking efforts. What better way to while away those idle days? But have these behaviours compounded the issues?

What will we, your doctors, find as we emerge from this pandemic? As we all move forward into an uncertain future?

Human behaviour during the early days of the pandemic made me angry. I was enraged to the point of disbelief. Despite the grave warnings, the cavalier attitude displayed by some put others at risk.

If only they saw what I saw, knew what I knew. As a key worker, I was always fast-tracked to the front of the supermarket queue. We were all fastidious about wearing masks then. It was mandatory for a reason. As I gazed around the busy supermarket, looking at the risk takers, I sized them up for the breathing tubes they would no doubt need. I wondered if I ever would be rid of these thoughts. The horrors that awaited us in the Covid wards during the pandemic's first few weeks. Would they still haunt me? The young people who came in with breathing difficulties affected us more. We treated these young people as if they were a son, a daughter, a niece or a nephew. Still, we didn't discriminate against young, old, black, brown, or white; they were all critically ill and needed urgent care.

Who we treated first? Who needed us the most? These were the decisions we grappled with. I watched the veterans, the older, wiser physicians amongst us; some plucked out of retirement, others volunteering their precious time and expertise to this war. At times they were as flustered as we were. None of us knew what it was we were dealing with. We treated the symptoms with the medicines and the training we had and learned, but the combination of the unknown and the speed at which this new enemy struck caught us all off guard. When a co-worker fell, we felt this loss profoundly. For some, this was too much; their grief couldn't be contained.

Why them? Why not me?

It took every ounce of our strength to keep going, to keep donning those suits that shielded us from this invisible enemy.

We all still carry the burden of this war, just like any veteran does. Some will wear the physical scars as a reminder of those challenging times; others will repress the emotional scarring and may even go on to lead everyday lives again. While those who were left deeply traumatised will need all the help and support they can get.

I celebrated my fiftieth birthday late. Covid delayed this celebration. As the pressure on the health system eased, restrictions were lifted, coinciding nicely with the start of summer. The weather continued to be pleasant. Progress looked good on the vaccine roll-out plan, and the collective mood of the nation was improving. The need to reach out to family and friends was overwhelming. A social but distancing street party is what it became. It was enough.

Christian arranged it all. He knows me well, better than anyone. I'm lucky. He fits so well into my network now. It didn't always used to be this way. When we first met, our differences seemed insurmountable. We were both products of a society seeped in prejudice. It would have been so easy to become a part of the spectacle. Instead, we both were open to the possibilities. My education cut a path through discrimination. The more I learned, the braver I felt, and the braver I felt, the more risks I took. It took a while before he noticed me at the hospital where we both worked. Such was his ability to see the person and not the packaging. At first, his world only overlapped mine in the ICU and patient wards. I admired his self-assurance and his confidence. He carried himself well and had good people skills. Unlike a few of his colleagues, he took the time to listen. His head would drop to his shoulder, and he would brush away the blond fringe that flopped over his face with the back of his hand. You'd then find yourself the sole focus of his piercing blue eyes. As a result, he was extremely popular with patients and staff alike.

He still moves this freely in any situation. I know he carries this sense of belonging into the world outside the walls of our home. His birthright affords him this freedom. My freedom feels less than out there. I shine bright in my spaces, home and hospital, where I am more open and contribute freely. Out there, in public, my light is dimmer. I move around with less self-assurance. I feel myself becoming smaller, my gaze lowering. This unconscious projection of peace and harmony speaks of a willingness to comply. When did I start feeling this way? When the only choices were compliancy or activism. Without being party to the insanity, do I play safe, or do I rise up? At times I've had to push back and verbally lash out, and for this, I'm the one that's judged harshly. So I live a dual existence. Please don't patronise me, don't label me.

Even in those troubled times, Christian didn't see colour. He only saw the unfairness. In our first proper encounter, he came to my defence in a café where I had repeatedly asked for a reheat of my coffee. All it took was a look from him, and the server and I were silenced. A hot coffee soon followed. Once we started talking, there was no stopping us. This connection felt genuine; it felt deep. Those first dates were passionate; we gave and received pleasure equally, but I also revealed my vulnerability—the gravity of which he will never truly understand.

Years later, I reminded him about that incident in the coffee shop; he claims there was no look. That proves my point; his mere white male presence was enough to spark action. Over the years, we have experienced many such moments. I'm grateful that he tries to understand why they deeply affect me. He now knows the indifference that I display in public masks the apprehension I sometimes feel. I have a deep sense of love for him, especially when he calls out any abusive behaviour. Let's just say that his actions make him even more desirable. But he will never truly understand.

It was hard work and strength of mind at school that rewarded me with a medical school scholarship. My mother's joy knew no bounds. She framed the acceptance letter, which took pride of place in her sitting room. She knew how much being a doctor meant to me and had been concerned that this dream would not become a reality through lack of funds.

Having successfully navigated the pitfalls of puberty, friendships, sexual relationships and the institution that was school, my awakening came. University presented new challenges. I walked in grounds and corridors where none of my ancestors had trodden.

The buildings were rich with a heritage and a culture that was so foreign to me. Although they carried the legacies of slavery and the spoils of exploitation, they also filled me with excitement and hope. I had the opportunity to rewrite the script. In the next wave of graduates, I could ensure that my people were represented; and I did. I passed with a first and looked forward to joining a hospital where I could finally begin to practice what I'd been learning for five long years. I worked in different specialities as a junior doctor, but the accident and emergency ward drew me. It was here that I genuinely felt I could have influence. As an emergency room doctor, you diagnose, stabilise and treat each patient. The breadth of clinical experience this gave me ensured that I grew in confidence. In peak periods, the pressure was immense. I endeavoured to approach each case with a fresh perspective and an open mind. Senior colleagues constantly reminded us *'patients are people, not statistics.*

Hungry for experience and without any romantic attachments back then, I had the freedom to work in different hospitals nation-wide. When I was first introduced to Christian, he was a consultant physician at the time and my supervisor. I wasn't sure if he even noticed me before then. He was definitely on my radar! As a now skilled junior, pending my final certificate of completion, I knew that my knowledge and confidence singled me out in assessments and supervised rounds. I'm unsure what he first noticed: my long braids, my arrogant certainty, or my razor-sharp mind. I like to think it was all of the above.

Bella was destined to work in A&E. She had the skills, experience, and, more importantly, the right instincts. She aced all her assessments. I sensed her desire to do well and be recognised for her ability.

I was determined to stand out for the right reasons. I could tell I came across as pushy and a know-it-all. I was driven by my desire to be the best. It sometimes felt like it was the only way anyone noticed the doctor, not my colour. They did start to take me seriously. If my peers saw me as competitive, then it meant that they thought I was a worthy adversary. I was okay with that.

Bella's confidence made her stand out. She carried herself with dignity and possessed such style. I soon noticed the attractive woman that she was. I found myself thinking about her a lot. And not always in a professional capacity. In a not-so-subtle way, I asked her colleagues where she hung out. Turns out she worked such long hours and practically lived at the hospital, only popping out occasionally to grab a decent cup of coffee.

A safe pair of hands is what I was known for being. Arrogant certainty then, in those scary times, was what was needed. My instincts served me well. We were a good team fighting this invisible virus. Our success stories were marked with joyful muffled cheering and clapping as our patients 'ran the gauntlet.' Discharged from the ward, avoided the morgue, and released back to their families. I counted the days until my release from the granny flat back into the family home.

Thinking back to when Christian and I first moved in together. Our demanding jobs and work schedule meant we had little time to enjoy this cohabitation. The tiny city flat, with its noisy plumbing, was an oft-neglected love nest because we spent so much time at the hospital. Our social life was non-existent due to the disparity of our schedules and the long hours we worked. Yet we endured. The love was true, and the sacrifices were worth it for those shared moments of abandoned joy.

When I finally met Christian's Scottish parents, they were kind and welcoming. Although I suspected they thought I was a fad that he'd eventually tire of. They spoke unapologetically about the type of women he had dated in the past and the connectedness of those families. The family photo albums showed how far from the usual type he had strayed.

Bella was shocked at the paleness of my life before her. I reminded her that we had often holidayed in the Caribbean as a family. She joked that it must have been a relief to return to 'the land of the pale' because of how light-toned we all were. I told her how much I loved being part of the collective consciousness of the island communities. They lived and worked together and seemed to breathe as one. Their spirit of togetherness is what our family enjoyed seeing. Lessons that the inhabitants of this 'land of the pale' could learn from.

The struggle to place this single-parent-raised, sometimes loud, singular Black woman in their reserved, traditional, and posh world was real. My 'middle-class' background had given me a home, love, state-funded education and a fair chance at a decent job, but this is where those similarities ended. Christian's 'middle-class' upbringing gave him wealth, status, private schooling, social acceptance and a passport to freedom. Throughout our courtship, and yes, that's what it was with him; good old-fashioned courting, he got to know me and, by extension, my family and community. He likened it to the clan culture of the Scottish highlands. My cultural education began at the same time.

As an interracial couple, we attracted attention. Whispers accompanied looks, which made me feel exposed and vulnerable. Chris's response was merely to smile and greet the perpetrators. It was usually the last comeback they expected. I, on the other hand, chose to withdraw into myself. I felt that if we were to be judged based solely on the colour of our skin, then I would ignore these offenders. They ceased to exist. Sometimes these differences in beliefs and judgments played out a little too close to home. Our respective families and their differing worlds became a catalyst for many upsetting moments. It took a long time to dispel the notion that I was with him to elevate my status. My people betrayed me by questioning my motives for being with a White man. As if choosing him over a Black man was a form of disloyalty. It took me a long time to put aside the hurt these remarks caused. Christian tried his best to empathise, but he could never truly understand my discomfort or the rage it sometimes invoked. Where work gave me a sense of purpose and invigorated me, harbouring these family and social resentments left me physically and mentally exhausted. Something was bound to shift.

But there was hilarity too. The laughter was good for my soul. Christian's attempts at getting to know my family by challenging them on the dancefloor, were hysterical. His aerobic gyrations certainly matched the energy of the room, if not the rhythm and bass of the music. Early celebrations were also a minefield of emotions, as our approaches were hugely different. For Christian, birthdays were always quiet, family-only celebrations. I used to wonder if they had any friends at all. It was the opposite for me. These were hearty celebrations, and guests came from far and wide. *I didn't realise your entire family came over on the Windrush. How will we accommodate all these people?* Any perceived dig at my culture brought out the worst in me. It would take many fights to work out that he was genuinely perplexed at these events and meant no harm.

We agreed to face each difficult moment with respect, tolerance and a pinch of humour. So it was how we successfully brought those cultures together on our wedding day. Early planning stages were reasonably uneventful, with the choice of church and venue being the only stumbling block. Christian's family lived in a beautiful historical village and were hellbent on us getting married in their local chapel, as they and their ancestors had done for years before. I belonged to the Baptist church and wanted the rituals and energy of the community spirit to prevail. Ultimately, we compromised and had a gospel choir present at the service and reception. I was delighted to see how the men in my bridal party embraced the wearing of morning suits. The shock and panic on the faces of some of the groom's party were equally delightful during those rousing choral moments. Throughout the day, we caught snippets of conversations that made us smile knowingly.

They make such a striking couple.

Yes, we were a striking couple, tall and short, fair and dark, and in love!

They will make beautiful children, all the colours of the rainbow.

We had no plans to have children soon. We were both committed to our profession and wanted to progress as far as possible.

Bella will follow Christian and specialise. Like him, she is ambitious.

Of course, I wanted more for myself and my people. I wanted to be a role model for young people in my ethnic group. *Bella will do what Bella will do!*

Christian will be happy with his exotic bride.

We made each other happy, and, at that moment, that's all that mattered. We agreed that this new marital partnership would never be limited or restricted by the ambition and desires of the individual. Our combined strength came from our happiness.

Christian is a lucky man!

As was I!

The stresses of work continued long after the wedding was over. For a while, we even found ourselves working at different hospitals. The split locations put a lot of pressure on our relationship. These choices had a significant impact on the way we socialised, slept, ate and functioned. Ready meals and snacking became my downfall again. As the years passed, the pounds piled on, and I was conscious that my health sometimes suffered. My head knew what needed to be done, but my heart was not in it. Christian knew how much pressure I was under and could be appropriately sympathetic or supportive. He saw me ride this weighty rollercoaster of shame, acceptance and change. But, having never had any problems with weight management, he could only be a silent observer of my journey.

I'm back in the Covid ward, where the problem of excess weight further complicated how this virus played out. I didn't need numbers or stats to work out that while this virus did not discriminate, it was the elderly, the vulnerable, the impoverished, and the obese that it hit the hardest. I saw these patients fighting for their lives. It was a messy war, one that stripped away all dignity. Nurses and attendants were busy mopping bodily fluids, checking ventilators, administering medication, and comforting those afraid. As I briefed doctors and checked patients' charts, I was sure that the smells that permeated the wards then would stay with everyone who survived this. It would forever invoke memories of the pain, the fear, and the discomfort in both the minds of patients and staff alike.

So different to the associations of the aromas that welcomed me back to a post in a hospital in Birmingham. Here the smells were associated with a much longed for home coming that spoke of exciting and new possibilities. There was a bit of resistance to our moving there. Christian thought it would be harder for him to feel accepted into a predominantly Afro-Caribbean neighbourhood. Selfishly, he also felt that our precious time together would be diluted, along with the demands of family and friends. Despite these initial reservations, he knew how much this move meant to me. It brought me back to my Mum, but most importantly, it brought me home. He was wrong on both counts. His acceptance was unconditional, and having the community's safety net gave us the freedom to be authentic. So it was fortuitous that after a minor health scare, he could scale back on his working hours, to manage his stress levels better. We both agreed that it was in his best interests to leave the demands of the hospital and instead accept a role as a clinical lecturer in Academia. This new shift in our home life meant he raised the subject of having a child. This idea soon became a reality with Chris working more predictable hours and potentially more present to raise a child. We'd finally considered all the pros and cons. I was thirty-eight and now firmly established as a consultant. Having a child this late took careful consideration on my part. My new role was even more demanding, and my weight was not ideal, so there were risks involved. Having been on the weight on, weight off rollercoaster over the years, I knew I could shed the pounds quickly by joining a local slimming club. All I needed was the support and accountability of a group. It never occurred to me to do this on my own. I'd always relied on their simplistic approach of telling *me what to eat and when to eat it.* With Christian's pledged support, operation weight-for-baby began in earnest.

I've watched Bells battle her weight over the years. As a medical professional, you'd think she'd know what to do, but like most people, stress, lifestyle, being time-poor and eating on the run mean risk and risky behaviours.

As a doctor, I know I should lead by example. For goodness' sake, I'm constantly telling my overweight and obese patients that losing weight starts with a choice. Instead of making excuses, ask instead, am I in control or not? This mental gear change is often enough to spark action. Christian operates differently.

She's always saying how easy it is for me. I know that my metabolism is different to hers. I'm also a tall male body, unlike her short female body. I could be on dangerous grounds here, but I think I'm a bit more aware of portion sizes, whereas she's not.

My body behaves differently from Chris's body. I am not a little man, so I cannot mimic his eating behaviours and choices. He loves his carbs yet is careful with the refined ones. He has willpower in abundance! I have cravings at various times of the month. Although I love fruit, my yearning for sugary treats will always triumph.

Chris forgets to eat. I cannot run on empty, as this affects my mood. Lately, more so. As I approach middle age, I feel less in control, not just with the cravings but also with how my body responds to them. I need to determine *what this changing body wants and how it behaves.* More exercise is what Christian suspects.

I've tried over the years, always unsuccessfully, to get Bells running with me. "Running? Why? Who is chasing you?" she'd jokingly remark while juggling her ample bosom.

This was perhaps the most complex shift in my mindset. I have never exercised knowingly and willingly. While I know the health benefits of exercise, I've never understood the enjoyment factor. Is it even possible to actually like exercise? Chris has always run and has taken part in a few race events. I watch his excitement build. Sometimes, I see the pain that training brings. I've always marvelled at the euphoria on completion. I'm curious about that unholy trinity of Anticipation-Pain-Elation that makes him keep going out there to do it all over again.

Bless her, though. She can be agonising when she's on a weight loss plan. I've learnt not to eat anything naughty in front of her. And when I say naughty, it pretty much covers everything! Brutal Bella is present until she conquers her cravings.

Probably for the best that Chris retreats to his study those first few days after I've joined a weight loss group; he will never understand the agony. He's never had a weight problem. He likes to tell my family that he still wears the same sized (and only ever mustard or red corduroy) trousers from school. That statement fails to impress, as they think he is starving and will immediately offer to cook traditional foods. That's the thing with my community, food and the social aspect of sharing meals, mainly traditional foods, is so important. I understand that all cultures celebrate with food. It's always going to mean so much more to my family. It represents comfort, love, healing and celebration. It's the glue that binds us. So why are we being harmed by food? Too many bad choices and not enough good ones? Bad practices? Not enough regulation? Mum learned how to manage her health by swapping some ingredients with healthier alternatives. It is possible to reverse some medical risks with good selections.

With operation weight-for-baby a success, and renewed desire, we started the baby-making process in earnest. Sex is a form of cardio, no? If so, Chris and I were set on getting into the best shape of our lives. Suddenly the exhaustion I used to feel as my day ended seemed to disappear when faced with the prospect of some rumpy-pumpy, as my husband calls it. I glowed. I couldn't help but reflect on these joyful feelings of making new life when faced with the harsh reality of losses almost on a weekly basis.

It didn't take long to fall pregnant. Oh, the joy, not just for Chris and I, but for Mum, my aunties and the rest of our extended families. Finally, they all agreed. It's been too long. It's a special feeling to be in the safe hands of colleagues for the duration of my pregnancy and for the birth itself. As medical staff, we have seen and know so much of what can go wrong. We know how to comfort, when to comfort and what to say to make patients feel at ease. I joked with the maternity staff that they had seen more of my bits than my husband had in those last few weeks leading up to the birth. Chris was by my side, holding my hand and whispering kind words. He wept as he was handed our son. With a look of awe and pure joy, he kept whispering: *I'm so proud of you. I love you, Bells. Thank you for our baby.*

The parental journey highlighted more differences in the way we raised our toddler. Sparing the rod, and spoiling the child was how I was raised. So naturally, any bad behaviour on my part had only one consequence, my mother's slipper—a light touch for sure, but one that stopped everyone in their tracks. My husband, growing up, did not get beaten at all, not once. Instead, he had the naughty step, leaving him to "contemplate the seriousness of his actions." I'm happy to introduce this form of discipline into our parenting, but I can't help cheekily baiting my mother-in-law, "What do you suppose Christian thought about while he sat there on the naughty step?"

How lucky we are to be surrounded by loving parents. They have welcomed this mixed-race baby and will fiercely protect him. I feel blessed to have been part of this journey of change and acceptance. I feel the love from my parents-in-law as they embrace me. I see their harsh assessment of those who criticise or question the colour of our baby's skin and his curly chestnut hair. I thank them for their unwavering support of my career choices and my decisions around raising our child.

We all agree there is no right and wrong way, and we always strive to be respectful, kind and fair.

Our boy thrives because of our united approach. By virtue of his upbringing and identity, he's also a person of privilege. I'm okay with that. Christian has also become firmly entrenched in our community. It keeps us all grounded. We give our son a healthy blend of Caribbean and British culture. He's ten now. He is a bright boy. Kind too, and very thoughtful. He knows that being respectful of his elders is essential. My mother has instilled that in him. Although with his cheeky grin and big hazel eyes, she spoils him too. Once again, a fruit slice or a sticky date and nut treat awaits him when he comes home. Although her health has improved significantly, Mum is frailer than before. Chris and I love having her live with us. She has taught our son so many Caribbean traditions. He even knows about his long-passed grandfather. He's often told that he has the same cheeky smile. We cannot wait to surprise Mum with another holiday to Jamaica. It's her eightieth birthday soon. So this time, it will include a visit to the town where she was born. Thus far, Covid has scuppered our plans. We will keep trying, though. It has got to happen.

After the shock of the pandemic and the relief that followed the vaccination programme, we returned to a new normal with the opportunity to play catch up. When the hospital offered post-Covid medical assessments, I signed up immediately with the rest of my staff. I wasn't particularly concerned as I felt blessed that I'd come through the worst of Covid relatively intact. So it was with surprise and concern that some of my health markers were flagged. Another revelation was that I was perimenopausal, which made sense of the hot flushes that had been bothering me lately. I know first-hand that the body we carry into our menopause is the body that is at risk for all the long-term consequences: weight gain, poor fitness levels, chronic stress, chronic inflammation and chronic illness. These are important to manage at any stage of life, but even more so as we age, especially for women like me, women my age.

I think back to the lady on the stretcher and how connected I felt to her then. Her death resonated with me. I could tell she was married, and so was possibly a mother too. My mind races back to when I was in self-imposed isolation and couldn't be with my family. I think of my son's tears each time we spoke through the glass. I recall Chris's words when I came home once with a sore throat and a temperature. *Please fight this with everything you've got, Bella. You are my world, my life. I need you. We need you.*

There's so much to be grateful for. My profession, my partner, my family, my friends and my community. Why wouldn't I fight for that?

Now, I just need to focus on my health risks and get this banging bod bikini ready.

Her name was Amani, the lady on the stretcher. I had asked my neighbour to reach out to her family. Despite the circumstances, I wanted them to know that she was treated well while in our care. Her husband called to thank me for being with her at the end.

All patients are people, not statistics!

| 9 |

Weathering and Future-proofing. Risk to Reward (part 1)

"Stay healthy," they cry.

It's all well and good saying stay healthy, but how exactly do we do that? We are ageing; we are transitioning. So we're unable to do the things we could in our twenties and thirties, not in the same way anyway. Who cares? We still feel relevant. Here's a thought. Why not just redefine what good health at this age means?

Surely it's not just a series of numbers, measures of function? That's clinical.

Healthy ageing is so much more.

But first, over to you, what are your measures of success when it comes to your overall health?

- Is it stepping on the scales and feeling in control?
- Still fitting into your wedding dress?
- Or feeling vital, with a sense of belonging?

Collectively these aspects should combine to give us a sense of balance for mind, body and spirit. You must have seen this mantra before. Wellness centres promote it all the time. But how exactly are they measuring it? And what are you left with?

I'll go first. I carry my burdens from a life lived so far. The death of a loved one, a couple of medical mishaps, maybe too much indulgence at times and even moments of woeful neglect, but that could be every woman.

I'm here now, future-focused, trying to do all the right things, and I'm happy to say that my path is smoothing. But it really isn't all about me.

Because joining me in today's webinar is my good friend, Joyce Getz, an authority on all that is female well-being, particularly what that means in middle age.

Joyce, tell us, how do you think you have weathered so far?

Thanks, Jayne, ha, I certainly was no saint either, but in the last decade, I've discovered that my body doesn't behave like before. I, too, have veered into treacherous grounds at times, making bad choices that have caused me to stumble and fall. I have learned that facets of life and health are dynamic and require constant fine-tuning and adjustment.

Jane: Do you mean the usual health hazards and risks that lie in store as women age?

Joyce: Yes, some hazards are avoidable, some predictable, and others, depending on the context, can be a mixture of both. Take stress, for example. Just enough can excite; too much can harm.

Jane: Agreed. How do we know when stress moves from excitement to causing harm?

Joyce: When the outcomes result in poor health or alarming health markers. That's when. Remember, middle-age is pivotal because we're in a perfect storm. We're facing life events of a more grave nature. So taking stock now is essential. First, let's talk about the layers we would already wear.

- Relationships identify us as lovers, partners, wives, mothers, sisters and daughters.
- Financial demands mean we are either self-employed, employers, employees or carers.
- As homemakers, we also function as cooks, taxi mums and social secretaries.

All of this while we continue to network in-and-outside of the home, often putting others' needs first with scant regard for ourselves.

Meanwhile, life events are happening around these roles. Some bring happiness and positivity to boost or enhance our lives. Others are major life events, like death or divorce. And if we haven't trumped already, here comes menopause and its societal taboos, along with the depletion of our protective oestrogen.

Jane: Ah, yes! That magical, hormonal balm helps safeguard our brain, heart, muscle & bone mass and keeps our mood in check. Let's not forget what it means for our sex life!

Joyce: Unsurprisingly, we carry more physical and emotional baggage than before. If we feel burdened, it's time to lighten the load and **buck the menopause**.

Jane: Oops, you've dropped the F-bomb there, Joyce!

Joyce: No, on the contrary, I mean let's do something about it.

Jane: I agree wholeheartedly. My listeners will know about riding the oestrogen wave and what that means for women's health. We covered that in an earlier podcast.

As life events and stressors start ramping up in middle age, the energy on the 'battery pack' is running low, revealing a plethora of emotional responses as we navigate our way forward. So what does that mean for us in the next decade or two? Stress levels are rising too, and if our health risks are increasing, wouldn't we want to keep checking these risks as often as we can?

Joyce: Most people are aware that their stress levels are on the increase. I wonder how many link it immediately to inflammation of the worst kind - *Chronic Inflammation*. Anxiety, depression, digestive issues, headaches, muscle tension and pain, sleep problems, weight gain, and memory and concentration impairment; these symptoms may be stress related. Either way, it begins with a release of stress hormones.

Jane: Those symptoms and conditions can so easily be attributed to menopause too. That's precisely why we need to take this seriously now.

Joyce: Absolutely. And on the more serious end of this spectrum, heart disease, heart attack, high blood pressure, and strokes are all stress related.

Jane: So it's stress that increases the risk of many physical and mental health problems. I know this is serious, but let's address this in a less than serious manner.

Joyce: Having tuned in to ALL your previous podcasts Jane, I'm all ears.

Jane: Generally, women come in all shapes and sizes—Apples, Pears, Celery's etc. Our body shape, in addition to many other health markers, is what the medical world uses to assess health risks.

Joyce: Taking a more holistic approach, Jane and I will first identify those risk factors that affect women in their middle years. But before we do so, we need to think about the women we represent. What they feel and what the medical practitioners see.

Jane: Of course we cannot invite 'everywoman' into my studio, so instead, we will create our own avatars. These avatars will find themselves traversing their health risk zones depending on the life events in play. How they behave and the choices they make, will either keep them safe, or they will find themselves on dangerous grounds.

Joyce: Dangerous or treacherous grounds indeed. Chronic stress, both physical and mental, is what we call this RED zone.

Jane: Are you ready to play the game of risk, Joyce? But not as you know it, because this is women's health Risk2Reward®

Joyce: Let's jump straight in.

Jane: To my listeners and viewers, Joyce and I will illustrate the game with our fictional characters or avatars in typical scenarios. We will play these characters individually for our listeners' clarity and understanding. The rules of the game become clearer as we start and progress with the first avatar before bringing the second into play.

(BTM: You will find more information about the rules of the game at the back of the book.)

So with that, my avatar is pear-shaped, and we'll call her Pear, while Joyce's avatar is called Apple.

Lady Pear
Aged 40
5ft 1 or 1.5m
63 kg/ 10 stone/140 lb
BMI 28
Waist / hip ratio 0.74
Activity level:
Low

Lady Apple
Aged 40
5ft 3 or 1.6m
63 kg/ 10 stone/140 lb
BMI 25
Waist / hip ratio 0.84
Activity level:
Moderate

Jane: Pear, aged forty, has a BMI indicating that she's in the overweight category of the spectrum. Her Waist-Hip ratio suggests low risk. She starts in the yellow zone. Her score represents a low health risk. Let's start by rolling the die that represent Ageing in years, number of Life Events and the number of Behavioural Hazards.

Joyce: So should we think of a random selection of life events and we choose the Behavioural Hazards or lifestyle choices that the avatar has in play at any time.

Jane: That's correct Joyce. The LE (life events) cards, the ER (emotional responses) cards and the BH (behavioural hazards) cards sit alongside the board which represents life's journey.

Without further ado, let's see what the first move on the board is for my avatar Pear.

1st dice roll = 2; Move forward 2 year(s) in age

2nd dice roll = 2; Random Selection 2 Life Event(s)

Based on LE cards in play, choose Emotional Response(s)

3rd dice roll = 5; Choose 5 Behavioural Hazard(s)

Age & Metrics		Green Zone	Yellow Zone	Amber Zone	Red Zone
Age	40+2yrs				
BMI	28		28		
Waist Hip Ratio	0.74		0.74		
Existing Health Conditions	None				
Life Events (LE)					
CARD 1: Relationship Betrayal (Other)					
CARD 2: Relationship Breakdown					
Emotional Responses (ER)					
Positive					
Negative			Fear, Shame	Sadness	Anger
Behavioural Hazards (BH)					
Behavioural Hazard (BH) in play			1. Saturated Fat; 2. Refined Carbohydrates; 3. Active Level (Low)	4. Smoking 5. Salt in excess	
with Associated Risks/Rewards (AR)			1. Heart Disease; 2. Diabetes; 3. Obesity Related & Heart Disease	4. Lung Disease 5. Hypertension	
Decision time		<----------------Walk Tall or Stumble Fall---------------->			

Pear Move 1

Jane: Pear, now two life years on. At first glance, into the deep we go—a breakdown of her relationship, possibly due to that betrayal. So the position of the ER cards is perfectly understandable. Anger is the dominant emotion and potentially the most damaging, which explains where it ends up. It definitely speaks of a betrayal with a loss of control.

Joyce: So, what else is going on?

Jane: A handful of Behavioural Hazard cards are in play here. Looking at these with their risk placement, here are my assumptions.

I'm guessing she uses smoking as a crutch and will reach for processed food when she feels unbalanced—perhaps looking for instant gratification. Is her mind possibly troubled with thoughts such as 'forgive or forget' and 'stay or go'?

Joyce: Strong emotions can do that! Reaching for whatever gives you comfort. The naughtier, the better! Hers is a classic case of feeding one's anger. I have helped women in similar situations where the overriding thought is, "sod it, what does it matter if the figure goes." Yet another way of pushing the errant partner out. *(Susie Orbach)*

Jane: It's a passive way of sticking two fingers up. We're all guilty of it. We know that self-sabotage doesn't punish the partner. If anything, it makes you feel worse.

Will this be a Walk Tall or Stumble and Fall moment for her?

1st dice roll = 1; Move forward 1 year(s) in age

2nd dice roll = 1; Random Selection 1 Life Event(s)

Based on LE cards in play, choose Emotional Response(s)

3rd dice roll = 6; Choose 6 Behavioural Hazard(s)

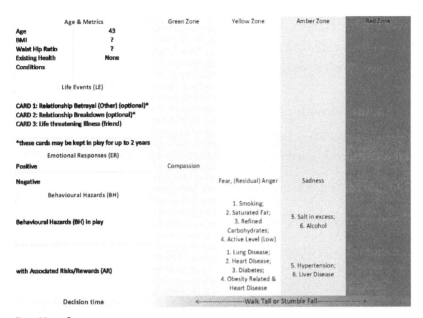

Age & Metrics		Green Zone	Yellow Zone	Amber Zone	Red Zone
Age	43				
BMI	?				
Waist Hip Ratio	?				
Existing Health Conditions	None				
Life Events (LE)					
CARD 1: Relationship Betrayal (Other) (optional)*					
CARD 2: Relationship Breakdown (optional)*					
CARD 3: Life threatening illness (friend)					
*these cards may be kept in play for up to 2 years					
Emotional Responses (ER)					
Positive		Compassion			
Negative			Fear, (Residual) Anger	Sadness	
Behavioural Hazards (BH)					
			1. Smoking;		
			2. Saturated Fat;		
Behavioural Hazards (BH) in play			3. Refined Carbohydrates;	5. Salt in excess; 6. Alcohol	
			4. Active Level (Low)		
			1. Lung Disease;		
			2. Heart Disease;		
with Associated Risks/Rewards (AR)			3. Diabetes;	5. Hypertension; 6. Liver Disease	
			4. Obesity Related & Heart Disease		
Decision time		<------------------Walk Tall or Stumble Fall------------------>			

Pear Move 2

Jane: Another year on, and another life event added. Her friend's illness will have an impact and remember; there is still the emotional legacy of the drama from the life events in the play previously.

Joyce: If Pear's close friend is female and of a similar age, statistically speaking, she's probably been diagnosed with breast cancer. If so, this friend would have been advised to rally her support team, which makes Pear party to the experience and the medical advice given. Perhaps this is why her smoking hazard level moves from the moderate to the low-risk zone. Have you noticed the alcohol hazard in play?

Jane: Yes, in the amber zone, indicating she exceeds 14 units per week.

Jane: Perhaps a lack of knowledge? I chose to keep the previously played LE cards in play because I suspect there will be residual emotional baggage. To top it all, she also carries the extended emotions linked to her friend's illness. I wonder if this is a pivotal moment in Pear's life to make personal lifestyle adjustments.

Joyce: We'll have to wait and see.

Another move for Pear.

1st dice roll = 2; Move forward 2 year(s) in age

2nd dice roll = 2; Random Selection 2 Life Event(s)

Based on LE cards in play, choose Emotional Response(s)

3rd dice roll = 7; Choose 7 Behavioural Hazard(s)

Age & Metrics		Green Zone	Yellow Zone	Amber Zone	Red Zone
Age	45				
BMI	?				
Waist Hip Ratio	?				
Existing Health Conditions	None				
Life Events (LE)					
CARD 1: Relationship Betrayal (Self)					
CARD 2: Relationship Strain					
Emotional Responses (ER)					
Positive		Pleasure, Excitement			
Negative				Guilt, Shame, Anxiety	
Behavioural Hazards (BH)					
Behavioural Hazards (BH) in play		1. Saturated Fat; 2. Refined Carbohydrates; 3. Active Level (Moderate); 4. Perimenopause (Somatic)	5. Smoking	6. Sexual Health; 7. Alcohol	
with Associated Risks/Rewards (AR)		1. Heart Disease; 2. Diabetes; 3. Improved Fitness/Fat Burn/Injury; 4. Discomfort Levels (Low) per MRS	5. Lung Disease	6. STD/Pregnancy; 7. Liver Disease	
Decision time		<-----------------Walk Tall or Stumble Fall----------------->			

Pear Move 3

Joyce: Gosh, what a turn of events! It would appear that relationship stress is ongoing. This time she's the guilty party. The emotional responses suggest she's swinging from pleasure to guilt. Perhaps a vengeful act for her partner's prior misdemeanours? Or an opportunity presenting itself when she was feeling vulnerable? Either way, she has acquired a further hazard and a corresponding risk - her sexual health. Her alcohol consumption remains the same. But on a positive note, look at where the usual suspects sit. Green zone on her nutrition means she appears to have a better handle on her food choices, *and* she's more active. Mm, what could be the cause of this increase in her activity level, I wonder?

Jane: Oi, oi! She's being naughty. Maybe the guilt will come from dealing with the consequences of being caught out, the possibility of having contracted an STD, or even an unwanted pregnancy. Perhaps that's why her shame and anxiety levels are high.

Joyce: Interestingly, STDs are a very real problem in midlife—a consequence of older adults divorcing and changing partners in this digital dating age. Lack of precaution or a reluctance to use barrier methods are just two causes I hear frequently.

Jane: At this age, you'd think we'd know better. It will be interesting to see if feeling desired has made her shake off the pounds.

Joyce: Have you spotted early signs of menopause yet?

NHS HEALTH CHECK: Aged 45 (BMI = 26; Waist Hip Ratio = 0.73; Existing Health Condition = None)

1st dice move = 3; Move forward 3 year(s) in age

2nd dice roll = 2; Random Selection 2 Life Event(s)

Based on LE cards in play, choose Emotional Response(s)

3rd dice roll = 6; Choose 6 Behavioural Hazard(s)

Age & Metrics		Green Zone	Yellow Zone	Amber Zone	Red Zone
Age	48				
BMI	26		26		
Waist Hip Ratio	0.73		0.73		
Existing Health Conditions	None				
Life Events (LE)					
CARD 1: Change in Job/Role					
CARD 2: Fledging Child					
Emotional Responses (ER)					
Positive		Relief, Joy			
Negative			Sadness	Self doubt, Sense of panic	
Behavioural Hazards (BH)					
Behavioural Hazards (BH) in play		1. Saturated Fat; 2. Refined Carbohydrates	3. Smoking; 4. Active Level (Low); 5. Alcohol	6. Perimenopause (Somatic)	
with Associated Risks/Rewards (AR)		1. Heart Disease; 2. Diabetes	3. Lung Disease; 4. Obesity Related & Heart Disease; 5. Liver Disease	6. Discomfort Levels (Moderate) per MRS	
Decision time			<-------------------Walk Tall or Stumble Fall------------------->		

Pear Move 4

Jane: So she did make positive changes on the nutrition front. Her BMI has gone down, and it looks like she's dodged the bullet of STDs.

Joyce: But her waistline is thickening. Mmm …

Jane: The usual life events in play here. Job role change and a fledging child can be experienced positively and negatively. They bring mixed emotional cards to the table. If her job role change is positive and the end of her full-time mother role is sad, then potentially, her risk levels are balanced, helped enormously by reducing her alcohol consumption. The only disruptor with this picture is the Perimenopause now playing out in the Amber zone.

Joyce: Looking at this move, Pear is in a good space. That is, until her perimenopause presents itself. Somatic, as we know, are those symptoms relating to the body. Flushes, palpitations, and joint and muscle aches in this zone indicate moderate to high discomfort levels. Life events now start to unfurl against this backdrop. She may be attributing those ERs of self-doubt and sense of panic to her change of circumstances, whereas it could be down to the hormonal storm that brews beneath the surface. From here on, the health risks associated with smoking may be amplified. Her behaviour might be the same, but the risk levels will increase. Once again being a smoker, studies show that could fast-track her into an early menopause.

Pear is in play again.

1st dice roll = 2; Move forward 2 year(s) in age

2nd dice roll = 3; Random Selection 3 Life Event(s)

Based on LE cards in play, choose Emotional Response(s)

3rd dice roll = 8; Choose 8 Behavioural Hazard(s)

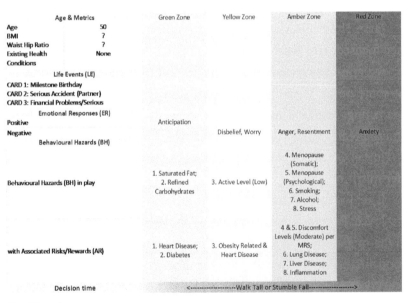

Age & Metrics		Green Zone	Yellow Zone	Amber Zone	Red Zone
Age	50				
BMI	?				
Waist Hip Ratio	?				
Existing Health Conditions	None				
Life Events (LE)					
CARD 1: Milestone Birthday					
CARD 2: Serious Accident (Partner)					
CARD 3: Financial Problems/Serious					
Emotional Responses (ER)					
Positive		Anticipation			
Negative			Disbelief, Worry	Anger, Resentment	Anxiety
Behavioural Hazards (BH)					
Behavioural Hazards (BH) in play		1. Saturated Fat; 2. Refined Carbohydrates	3. Active Level (Low)	4. Menopause (Somatic); 5. Menopause (Psychological); 6. Smoking; 7. Alcohol; 8. Stress	
with Associated Risks/Rewards (AR)		1. Heart Disease; 2. Diabetes	3. Obesity Related & Heart Disease	4 & 5. Discomfort Levels (Moderate) per MRS; 6. Lung Disease; 7. Liver Disease; 8. Inflammation	
Decision time		<-------------------Walk Tall or Stumble Fail------------------>			

Pear Move 5

Jane: Blimey! Look at these cards. Wow, it's ramped up! What's going on? The accident is a curve ball, and the financial fallout is perhaps a direct consequence. Why the anger and resentment, though? Maybe the partner did something foolish and could have avoided the severity of the injury and its implications. Who knows?

Joyce: What a leap Jane. AssumptionsRus! Where are you hiding that crystal ball?

Jane: Intuition maybe, and besides, we've seen it all before with her. She's back in the red zone with anxiety. And look at what she's doing. In the Amber zone, she's drinking and smoking. She is a lady under pressure! Her stress card mirrors her risk level.

Joyce: Agreed. It's her stress levels that I would be more concerned about. It's not only the life events because here we are, and as predicted, she's in full-blown menopause, aged 48. It is a stumble-and-fall moment for her. How long she stays will determine her health outcomes.

Jane: Hold up. Maybe a pending milestone birthday will keep her focused. Her health may still be good, even though the amber or red zone behaviours may send her off to medical professionals at some point. Looking at her nutrition choices, she's still weight managing. And let's be honest, for some, it's vanity that rules. I was undoubtedly in the best shape at that age.

Joyce: Good point. In this instance, her vanity may help regulate her nutrition.

Jane: I wonder what's her gauge. Dress size or scale?

Joyce: Perhaps both. At a guess, I'd say she's turning to slimming clubs or fad diets. Traditional slimming methods tend to restrict food intake alone. Weight loss happens by creating a significant weekly food calorie deficit. But we know how hard that is to maintain. Rapid weight loss signals the brain that the body is in "famine mode", and we all have different responses when that happens. For some, when the regime ends, it means adding back the loss and more!

Jane: Classic yo-yo dieting. It works because it's targeted and has a specific deadline. In her case a fiftieth birthday.

Joyce: Yes, weight management needs a more joined-up approach. In a nutshell: Getting your head right, sticking to a balanced nutrition plan, moving more and having accountability along with the support of others.

Jane: But now, with menopause, as we know, the body doesn't behave in its usual way.

Joyce: Absolutely! We don't process sugar in the same way. Our body fat distribution is different, mainly around the trunk, and our metabolism slows down, so we have to work harder to achieve those same results. As a result, any sense of vulnerability is heightened, and possibly the sense of self and certainty is compromised. Perhaps that is why her Menopause (Psychological) card is in play too.

NHS HEALTH CHECK: Aged 50 (BMI 25; Waist Hip Ratio = 0.76; Menopause = Confirmed; Existing health conditions = None)

Jane: It's better than I thought. Her low-risk BMI and clean bill of health are reassuring.

Joyce: Indeed, however, there are still challenges ahead.

1st dice roll = 2; Move forward 2 year(s) in age

2nd dice roll = 1; Random Selection 1 Life Event(s)

Based on LE cards in play, choose Emotional Response(s)

3rd dice roll = 8; Choose 8 Behavioural Hazard(s)

Age & Metrics		Green Zone	Yellow Zone	Amber Zone	Red Zone
Age	52				
BMI	25	25			
Waist Hip Ratio	0.76		0.76		
Existing Health Conditions	None				
Life Events (LE)					
CARD 1: Financial Problems/Serious (Optional)*					
CARD 2: Life-threatening Illness (Partner)					
*these cards may be kept in play for up to 2 years					
Emotional Responses (ER)					
Positive					
Negative			Shock, Disbelief	Worry, Fear	Anxiety
Behavioural Hazards (BH)					
Behavioural Hazards (BH) in play				1. Saturated Fat; 2. Refined Carbohydrates; 3. Active Level (Minimal); 4. Postmenopause (Somatic) 5. Postmenopause (Psychological)	6. Smoking; 7. Alcohol; 8. Stress (Fight or Flight)
with Associated Risks/Rewards (AR)				1. Heart Disease; 2. Diabetes; 3. Obesity Related & Heart Disease; 4 & 5. Discomfort Levels (Moderate) per MRS;	6. Lung Disease; 7. Liver Disease; 8. Inflammation
Decision time			<------------Walk Tall or Stumble Fall------------>		

Pear Move 6

Jane: Two years after her fiftieth, the cards show her partner is at risk of dying. Another curveball. Another shock. Another accumulation of emotional and physical wear and tear.

Joyce: Indeed. None of us can know how to react until a crisis like this happens. She may not have had enough time to recover from the last blow. Alongside this is an hourglass of oestrogen time slowly running out.

Jane: The blows are happening repeatedly. She is just coping. Maybe it's a question of *how long you stumble and fall* rather than whether you do or don't.

Joyce: Let's be realistic. These free-falling (minus the parachute) moments can look and feel different for each person. When it feels like you're spinning out of control, experiencing severe levels of panic, and feeling utterly helpless, that would be the time to reach out and get professional help.

Jane: Let's discuss the Stress (fight or flight) card. What does a red zone placement mean for Pear?

Joyce: In medical speak, her autonomic nervous system has been triggered. She may be sleepless and experiencing constant fear and panic, ramped up by the level of drinking and smoking. It looks like her nutrition is on the back burner. That is why her risks have crept into the Red Zone. And don't forget, having started early, she's postmenopausal now.

Jane: Is it stress or the menopause that's put her there?

Joyce: Probably both. It's easy to attribute worry, fear and anxiety to life events. The events feel tangible, making their emotional responses appropriate and socially acceptable. But these same emotions can also be attributed to the menopause. Out of context, they can easily be misinterpreted and misunderstood by all in her social and cultural environment, not least her. Does that make sense, Jane?

Jane: I think so. Where would that leave her without those life events in play to pin her emotional state on? Confused is the answer. So maybe her stress is not a case of either or, but rather a combination. Poor Pear!

I think she needs help. Time for the **Wild Card** now, the panic attack.

Joyce: That means she has to go off to the **Medical Experts**.

NHS HEALTH VISIT: (Diagnosis = Depressive Disorder so Antidepressants prescribed; BMI = 28; Waist Hip Ratio = 0.77)

Pear resumes play

1st dice roll = 3; Move forward 3 year(s) in age

2nd dice roll = 2; Random Selection 2 Life Event(s)

Based on LE cards in play, choose Emotional Response(s)

3rd dice roll = 8; Choose 8 Behavioural Hazard(s) + Diagnosis CARD (#9)

Age & Metrics		Green Zone	Yellow Zone	Amber Zone	Red Zone
Age	55				
BMI	28		28		
Waist Hip Ratio	0.77		0.77		
Existing Health Conditions	Depressive Disorder				
Life Events (LE)					
CARD 1: Wedding (Family Member)					
CARD 2: Parental Responsibility (Financial)					
Emotional Responses (ER)					
Positive		Pride, Anticipation, Joy			
Negative (Includes a 'Wild ER CARD')			Concern, Heartache	Low Sense of Self	Anxiety, Panic Attack
Behavioural Hazards (BH)					
Behavioural Hazards (BH) in play				1. Saturated Fat; 2. Refined Carbohydrates; 3. Active Level (Minimal); 4. Post-menopause (Psychological); 5. Weight Gain 6. Stress	7. Smoking; 8. Alcohol; 9. Depressive Disorder/Antidepressants
with Associated Risks/Rewards (AR)				1. Heart Disease; 2. Diabetes; 3. Obesity Related & Heart Disease; 4. Discomfort Levels (Moderate) per MRS; 5. Obesity Related & Heart Disease; 6. Inflammation	7. Lung Disease; 8. Liver Disease; 9. Sexual Dysfunction/Weight Issues
Decision time		<------------------Walk Tall or Stumble Fall------------------>			

Pear Move 7

Jane: Pear is a crucial player in this family wedding, explaining the positive emotional response. Her stress level has gone down.

Joyce: The antidepressants may have helped with that. She'll still need to be vigilant and review this prescription in the future.

Jane: Interesting to note also that her postmenopausal hazards have changed. The Somatic symptoms are no longer there.

Joyce: She's a few years on now. Using the Straw+10 study as a guide, it makes perfect sense, as any clinician will know. She's transitioning in this post-menopausal stage. Somatic symptoms have been known to recede, sometimes to be replaced by others.

NHS HEALTH CHECK: Aged 55 (BMI = 31; Waist Hip Ratio = 0.84; Existing Medical conditions = Depressive Disorder)

1st dice roll = 2; Move forward 2 year(s) in age

2nd dice roll = 4; Random Selection 4 Life Event(s)

Based on LE cards in play, choose Emotional Response(s)

3rd dice roll = 11; Choose 11 Behavioural Hazard(s) + Diagnosis CARD (#12)

Age & Metrics		Green Zone	Yellow Zone	Amber Zone	Red Zone
Age	57				
BMI	31			31	
Waist Hip Ratio	0.79		0.79		
Existing Health Conditions	Depressive Disorder				
Life Events (LE)					
CARD 1: Life-threatening illness (Partner)					
CARD 2: Relationship Strain					
CARD 3: Change to Financial Status					
CARD 4: Death of Partner					
Add a Calamity **Wild CARD** (Covid)					
Emotional Responses (ER)					
Positive					
Negative			Worry, Fear	Grief, Anxiety	Depressed, Lonely
Behavioural Hazards (BH)					
Behavioural Hazards (BH) in play			1. Smoking; 2. Post-menopause (Vasomotor)	3. Post-menopause (Psychological) 4. Saturated Fat; 5. Refined Carbohydrates; 6. Salt in excess	7. Post-menopause (Uro-Genital) 8. Active Level (Sedentary) 9. Alcohol; 10. Stress 11. Connectivity (Loneliness); 12. Antidepressants
with Associated Risks/Rewards (AR)			1. Lung Disease; 2. Discomfort Levels (Low) per MRS	3. Discomfort Levels (Moderate) per MRS; 4. Heart Disease; 5. Diabetes; 6. Hypertension	7. Discomfort Levels (Severe) per MRS 8. Obesity Related & Heart Disease; 9. Liver Disease; 10. Inflammation 11. Poor Physical & Mental Health; 12. Sexual Dysfunction/Weight Issues
Decision time			<----------------Walk Tall or Stumble Fall--------------->		

Pear Move 8

Jane: Yet another blow for Pear. She's clearly distressed. Life is not kind to her. Her partner's dreaded illness has likely returned and is now terminal. That would explain the financial concerns. She will need to play an active role in his care. Without the necessary buffering and resources, this character will be desperate. The cards alone are stacked against her. Her choices appear to be limited.

And on top of that, Covid strikes. These events alone point to the fact that she's on a collision course, and it doesn't get much worse than that unless the death card is played. But, oh no, there it is.

She would be forgiven for buckling under the enormity of such a grim situation. It would be so easy to lose a sense of self and self-care at this time.

Joyce: What an assault of life events. Her situation looks so desperate. But it can get worse. It could end with her premature death. Just look at her hazards in play and the risks they point to. Her health risks have compounded and may indicate chronic diseases in the near future. Unless she has the strongest of constitutions, she's destined to crash.

Jane: Her discomfort level in post-menopause has amplified further. The frequency and intensity of her Uro-Genital symptoms are in a severe category.

Joyce: Sadly that's unfortunate. It may not always happen that way though. In her case, urogenital symptoms can so easily be linked to the side effects of her medication or a lack of desire. Either way, it's bound to be uncomfortable.

Jane: Ouch! And we know there are treatments out there. Now is not the time for her to be a passenger in her life. Look at what has happened to the smoking card since the last play. Can you see that she is capable of taking control? She's either given it up or maybe trying hard to do so.

Joyce: That's good news. Although weight gain, sleeplessness, and irritability are among the many withdrawal symptoms and side effects, she reduces her risk of lung disease every month and every year by being smoke-free. The health benefits are felt immediately. Psychologically too, it proves that she can overcome unhealthy habits.

Jane: If she continues to actively look after herself, including being open to help from the medical professionals, a U-turn is possible. I want to remind our listeners that antidepressant prescriptions can be revisited as part of any future health checks.

Joyce: Because the CALAMITY card is now in play, Jane, you also get a MEDICAL card.

Jane: Ah yes, this is the perfect time to play her Medical Experts card. This will point her in the right direction.

Joyce: I feel we'll see her again in the future. She's a survivor. She still has a life to live.

Other new and exciting opportunities to explore, maybe even grandchildren. It's all there.

With Pear off the board, Apple now turns forty and is in play.

1st dice roll = 2; Move forward 2 year(s) in age

2nd dice roll = 3; Random Selection 2 Life Event(s)

Based on LE cards in play, choose Emotional Response(s)

3rd dice roll = 5; Choose 5 Behavioural Hazard(s)

	Age & Metrics	Green Zone	Yellow Zone	Amber Zone	Red Zone
Age	40+2yrs				
BMI	25	25			
Waist Hip Ratio	0.84		0.84		
Existing Health Conditions	Gestational Diabetes				
Life Events (LE)					
CARD 1: Post pregnancy (Geriatric, 1st child)					
CARD 2: End of Maternity leave					
CARD 3: Maintain Work/Life Balance					
Emotional Responses (ER)					
Positive		Joy, Relief			
Negative			Fear, Worry	Guilt	
Behavioural Hazards (BH)					
Behavioural Hazards (BH) in play		1. Refined Carbohydrates; 2. Active Level (Moderate)	3. Post Pregnancy Health; 4. Abdominal (Visceral) Obesity	5. Stress	
with Associated Risks/Rewards (AR)		1. Diabetes; 2. Improved Fitness/Fat Burn/Injury	3. & 4. Cardiovascular Disease & Diabetes	5. Inflammation	
Decision time		<----------------Walk Tall or Stumble Fall---------------->			

Apple Move 1

Jane: Apple begins her journey in the low-risk zone based simply on her BMI. However, her Waist Hip Ratio puts her in a different zone. What does that mean for this Avatar?

Joyce: With a low-risk BMI, another flag for Apple will be this ratio. Statistically, people carrying more weight around their middle face more health risks than those with more weight around their hips.

Jane: Fascinating. I wonder how many of us would recognise that?

Joyce: Continuing. Gestational diabetes, a pre-existing condition with her pregnancy, seems to be now resolved. This was a late-in-life first pregnancy. The emotional responses are usual with this event.

Jane: Not sure I like the term 'Geriatric pregnancy.' That aside, she will have the usual guilt and dilemma of returning to work and possibly leaving her baby in someone else's care.

Joyce: Apple's fear and concern about returning to work will be balanced by the joy and relief of overcoming the risks of having had a healthy baby this late.

Jane: Birthing produces both babies and guilt complexes. I hope that she is well supported on both home and work fronts.

Joyce: Yes, that's true. It's worth remembering that none of us get it entirely right. We just are trying our best.

1st dice roll = 3; Move forward 3 year(s) in age

2nd dice roll = 5; Random Selection 5 Life Event(s)

Based on LE cards in play, choose Emotional Response(s)

3rd dice roll = 4; Choose 4 Behavioural Hazard(s)

Age & Metrics		Green Zone	Yellow Zone	Amber Zone	Red Zone
Age	45				
BMI	?				
Waist Hip Ratio	?				
Existing Health Conditions	None				
Life Events (LE)					
CARD 1: Parental Responsibility (Early Years)*					
CARD 2: Job Promotion					
CARD 3: Change in Job/Role					
CARD 4: Discrimination - Jeopardy (Age)*					
CARD 5: Discrimination - Jeopardy (Female)*					
*these cards may be kept in play throughout					
Emotional Responses (ER)					
Positive		Proud, Confident, Supported, Self Actualisation			
Negative			Self doubt, Imposter Syndrome	Guilt	
Behavioural Hazards (BH)					
Behavioural Hazards (BH) in play		1. Active Level (Moderate);	2. Refined Carbohydrates 3. Weight Loss; 4. Stress;		
with Associated Risks/Rewards (AR):		1. Improved Fitness/Fat Burn/Injury	2. Diabetes 3. Malnutrition; 4. Inflammation		
Decision time		<----------- Walk Tall or Stumble Fall----------->			

Apple Move 2

Joyce: Gosh, what a busy hand. Several life events are in play at once—an interesting set of cards. On the one hand, promotion is something to be celebrated as it points to success, financial gains, and networking. On the other hand, however, the price of this could be added pressure and expectations, hence the imposter syndrome, not to mention the impact these events can have on family life.

Jane: You're making many assumptions there; job success doesn't always sit comfortably alongside the role of 'Super mum.'

Joyce: Does it ever? Most of my clients would echo that thought.

Jane: I've noticed that her intake of refined carbohydrates has increased. So why is the weight loss card in play? Typically, unhealthy food choices point to an increase in weight/BMI.

Joyce: Not necessarily so; it may be that she's generally eating too little. Unhealthy choices have crept in. Perhaps quick burn empty calorie choices as fuel. Plus, having a young child means she's moving around more than usual.

Jane: Yep, that sounds about right. Welcome to the Toddler Years.

Joyce: Let's talk about the double jeopardy discrimination cards. We don't know what they relate to exactly, but at a guess, I'd say, one - she's female, perhaps in the minority in her peer group, and two - possibly one of the oldest too. So she'd feel the pressure.

Jane: Hold on, let's look at those cards again. Let's assume that since her entry onto the board, her health has remained stable; she's secured a promotion and has remained a loving partner and mother. All the while, she was dealing with societal injustices. That's pretty impressive by anyone's standards.

Play continues with Apple.

NHS HEALTH CHECK: Aged 45 (BMI = 26; Waist Hip Ratio = 0.86; Existing Health Conditions: Pre-High Blood Pressure)

No medication is needed at this point—no other health concerns.

1st dice roll = 3; Move forward 3 year(s) in age

2nd dice roll = 3; Random Selection 3 Life Event(s)

Based on LE cards in play, choose Emotional Response(s)

3rd dice roll = 5; Choose 5 Behavioural Hazard(s) + Diagnosis CARD (#6)

Age & Metrics		Green Zone	Yellow Zone	Amber Zone	Red Zone
Age	48				
BMI	26		26		
Waist Hip Ratio	0.86			0.86	
Existing Health Conditions	Pre-High Blood Pressure				
Life Events (LE)					
CARD 1: Inequality Protest (BLM)					
CARD 2: Maintain Work/Life Balance					
CARD 3: Discrimination - Jeopardy (Age)*					
CARD 4: Discrimination - Jeopardy (Female)*					
CARD 5: Discrimination - Jeopardy (Ethnicity)*					
*these cards may be kept in play throughout					
Emotional Responses (ER)					
Positive		Supported			
Negative			Disappointment, Frustration, Disgust	Guilt, Anxiety	
Behavioural Hazards (BH)					
Behavioural Hazards (BH) in play		1. Active Level (Moderate)	2. Refined Carbohydrates	3. Abdominal (Visceral) Obesity 4. Stress (heightened fight/flight response); 5. Insomnia (sleeplessness & acute fatigue)	6. Pre-High Blood Pressure
with Associated Risks/Rewards (AR)		1. Improved Fitness/Fat Burn/Injury	2. Diabetes	3. Cardiovascular Disease & Diabetes 4. Inflammation & compromised immunity; 5. Mental & Physical health	6. Hypertension & Stroke
Decision time		<----------------Walk Tall or Stumble Fall---------------->			

Apple Move 3

Jane: Oh dear. These cards speak of a climate of discord. One shows a racial movement; the others point to discrimination, possibly in both the workplace and public life. These outcomes suggest she's a woman of colour. Joyce, would you like to drive this assessment?

Joyce: Absolutely! I'm going to do that firstly as a professional and secondly as a woman of colour myself. What do we know so far? Her child has just started school, so her pace of life will be different now. Based on her recent NHS health check, her BMI health risk is still low; however, with a slightly elevated blood pressure reading and her ethnicity, she will be moved into the following risk category of Moderate. Like many women at this age, she may be oblivious to perimenopausal symptoms. If indeed she has them.

Jane: Yes, she would easily mistake any flush or her sleeplessness for the upset of the current environment.

Joyce: Indeed. As a woman of colour, my second assessment recognises that the discrimination cards at play can bring out different emotional and physical responses that no one around her would notice. For example, if she is a professional woman, she would expect and receive respect, yet in the climate of the inequality protest, she would be regularly verbally abused, and her competence put into question by the slurs and the insults possibly directed her way. She would be bracing herself each day for that. As a result, she may find herself in a constant state of anxiety. Sleeplessness might follow with fatigue, headaches, infections, and general malaise. That's the usual outcome of inner turmoil.

Jane: But that's so unfair. Would she feel that there's nothing she can do about it?

Joyce: It is unfair, but we have coping strategies in place. By the time you get to our age, many are in play, and they become so automatic. That's one of the benefits of ageing. So any strategy to counter negativity is a good one.

Jane: I hear you, but what does that mean for our lady?

Joyce: She has to think safe and wise outcome rather than venting her spleen.

Jane: By not calling it out or letting it fester?

Joyce: It needs to come out! But best elegantly done. Festering or wear-and-tear is how your physiological and mental health is compromised. This melting pot of life events and its stressors can lead to **allostatic stress**—the low-lying, sinister drip, drip erosion of good health. So, call it if you must or find an exit route, and keep safe and healthy.

Jane: So allostatic stress, put simply, means bad health by stealth!

Let's see what her next move looks like.

1st dice move = 2; Move forward 2 year(s) in age

2nd dice roll = 2; Random Selection 2 Life Event(s)

Based on LE cards in play, choose Emotional Response(s)

3rd dice roll = 6; Choose 6 Behavioural Hazard(s) + Diagnosis CARD (#7)

Age & Metrics		Green Zone	Yellow Zone	Amber Zone	Red Zone
Age	50				
BMI	?				
Waist Hip Ratio	?				
Existing Health Conditions	Pre-High Blood Pressure				
Life Events (LE)					
CARD 1: Wedding (Family)					
CARD 2: Maintain Work/Life Balance					
CARD 3: Discrimination - Jeopardy (Age)*					
CARD 4: Discrimination - Jeopardy (Female)*					
CARD 5: Discrimination - Jeopardy (Ethnicity)*					
*these cards may be kept in play throughout					
Emotional Responses (ER)					
Positive		Joy			
Negative			Sensitive	Vigilant, Hurt	
Behavioural Hazards (BH)					
Behavioural Hazards (BH) in play		1. Active Level (Moderate)	2. Refined Carbohydrates	3. Abdominal (Visceral) Obesity 4. Stress (heightened fight/flight response); 5. Insomnia (sleeplessness & acute fatigue); 6. Perimenopause (Somatic)	7. Pre-High Blood Pressure
with Associated Risks/Rewards (AR)		1. Improved Fitness/Fat Burn/Injury	2. Diabetes	3. Cardiovascular Disease & Diabetes 4. Inflammation & compromised immunity; 5. Mental & Physical health 6. Discomfort Levels (Moderate) per MRS	7. Hypertension & Stroke
Decision time		<---------------Walk Tall or Stumble Fall--------------->			

Apple Move 4

Jane: That's quite a suite of cards in play. For many, what would usually be a happy occasion seems also to have triggered adverse emotions in Apple. Her triple jeopardy cards will follow her along this game of life.

Joyce: Yes. Along with all their associated hazards and risks. She may be sensitive to the often-unintentional negative comments and remarks. Her hypervigilance may have developed from constantly having to deal with the biases in her life. No matter how well she manages herself in these situations, the usual suspects will keep triggering her default emotional responses.

Jane: Hopefully, somewhere between her coping strategies and societal awareness of unconscious bias, she will find peace. Until then, her health risks lean towards the moderate zones. Since her last check, it would appear that she oscillates gently between the low-risk and medium-risk zones.

Joyce: Perimenopausal Somatic in play now with moderate discomfort levels, so no major concerns there.

1st dice roll = 2; Move forward 2 year(s) in age

2nd dice roll = 2; Random Selection 2 Life Event(s)

Based on LE cards in play, choose Emotional Response(s)

3rd dice roll = 7; Choose 7 Behavioural Hazard(s) + Diagnosis CARD (#8)

Age & Metrics		Green Zone	Yellow Zone	Amber Zone	Red Zone
Age	52				
BMI	28		28		
Waist Hip Ratio	0.89				0.89
Existing Health Conditions	High Blood Pressure				
Life Events (LE)					
CARD 1: Inequality Protest (George Floyd)					
CARD 2: Maintain Work/Life Balance					
CARD 3: Discrimination - Jeopardy (Age)*					
CARD 4: Discrimination - Jeopardy (Female)*					
CARD 5: Discrimination - Jeopardy (Ethnicity)*					
Add a Calamity Wild CARD (Covid)					
*these cards may be kept in play throughout					
Emotional Responses (ER)					
Positive		Compassion, Determination			
Negative			Sadness, Disbelief	Anger, Fear	Anxiety
Behavioural Hazards (BH)					
Behavioural Hazards (BH) in play		1. Active Level (Moderate to Vigorous)	2. Refined Carbohydrates	3. Abdominal (Visceral) Obesity 4. Acute Fatigue; 5. Perimenopause (Somatic) 6. Severe Migraines	7. Stress (heightened fight/flight response); 8. High Blood Pressure/Medicated
with Associated Risks/Rewards (AR)		1. Improved Fitness/Fat Burn/Injury/Exhaustion	2. Diabetes	3. Cardiovascular Disease & Diabetes 4. Mental (PTSD) & Physical health; 5. Discomfort Levels (Moderate) per MRS 6. Ischaemic strokes	7. Inflammation & compromised immunity; 8. Hypertension & Stroke
Decision time		<------------Walk Tall or Stumble Fall------------>			

Apple Move 5

NHS HEALTH CHECK: Aged 50 (Postponed until one year after the pandemic)

Jane: It would appear that this character has been sideswiped. We know that her stress levels were already elevated in the last two moves. Covid strikes and tips it into a different stratosphere. Oh, dear! She was in the driving seat and doing so well.

Joyce: This is a maelstrom scenario. A pandemic strikes at the same time she hits fifty. Menopausal symptoms continue their silent attack. Let's unpick the cards. It screams distress to me.

Jane: Agreed, and very loudly too.

Joyce: Acute fatigue, migraine, hypertension risk, PTSD...I wonder if Apple is a key worker and in the thick of it. Do you think she's attributing any of her symptoms and health complaints to either the Covid chaos or the Menopause? Would her health status even register at a time when she's in the thick of it?

Belated NHS HEALTH CHECK: (BMI = 28; Waist Hip Ratio = 0.89; Diagnosis = High Blood Pressure. Medication prescribed)

Jane: And there we have it. It's taken its toll. Her Blood pressure and BMI has elevated since her last check-in.

Joyce: Covid was the game changer for this character. She may have been too busy looking after others ahead of her health. Plainly, she's always driven her risks, and in a pre-pandemic situation, she would have acted on the hypertension risk sooner.

Jane: Covid interrupted everything, including that all-important milestone health check. I wonder how many of our listeners were 'blindsided' like this character. Especially at a time when health monitoring took a backseat as priorities shifted. We were all too busy just coping with the crisis.

Joyce: It was an incredible period. Time took on a new meaning. A surreal existence. I thought life would never be the same again, although it was worth remembering Maya Angelou, who said, "Every storm runs out of rain."

Jane: I love it; it's so true, though. Allowing us time to regroup and chart a new course forward. What a journey this has been for our players! By now, viewers will align their paths with these avatars' aspects. Perhaps pondering their possible pre-loads.

Joyce: Precisely. That has been the point of this game. As the players mid-lives unfolded, they collected more risks. Going into menopause and post-menopause when they did, suggested that they may have already been pre-loaded. Without any mitigation, they could potentially have been a ticking bomb.

Jane: Thank goodness they had professional check-ins and help along the way.

Joyce: Keep assessing your health risks; also, consider life stressors and your responses to them. Think about the safety net of support from relationships, social, cultural, and professional. Finally, think about the choices you make.

We'd like you all to WALK TALL.

Jane: This brings us to the end of the game of **Risk2Reward**® for these two avatars, Apple and Pear. They've served their purpose.

Please stay tuned for the podcast version of Weathering and Future-proofing Risk to Reward (part 2)

| 10 |

Weathering and Future-proofing. Risk to Reward (part 2)

Jane: Welcome back to Weathering and future-proofing from *Risk to Reward.* It's clear now that so many other aspects of your life affect your health risks.

Joyce: I agree. Good health is so much more than just a BMI score.

Jane: Do you mean the holistic approach? Of Mind, Body, and Soul? What many of us know.

Joyce: Yes, but not necessarily how you know it. And yes, as many wellness specialists do, we will start with the tangible metrics of the Body. Energy in (Nutrition) and Energy out (Movement). The Measurables. These two measurables or markers can be used to produce a Health indicator. Get your equation wrong, and the imbalance can tip you into a risky health zone over time. Get it right, and that direction changes towards safer zones where you start to reap the rewards.

Jane: When I think of energy in and energy out, I think of calorie counting as part of weight management. The outcome of success here spells vanity first before good health. Or is that just me?

Joyce: True, that's obvious for most. People understand rewards differently. Let's begin with six simple rewards: *Eating, Moving, Sleeping, Nature, Tribe,* and *Harmony.*

Jane: That's interesting. I've never really thought of these as rewards. I do most of these anyway, at least the first three.

Joyce: Many of us don't focus on the rewards specifically. When the indicator known as Health connects with our Self-esteem, another measurable domain, **BODY**, is created.

Jane: That makes sense. Body health *is* usually linked to self-esteem.

Joyce: Now that we've identified the domain (**BODY**), let's explore what the simple six rewards mean in this space:

- *Eating* means healthy eating, making good choices, feeding and fuelling the body
- *Moving* means moving for your heart health, striking a balance between resting, fat-burning, cardio, and peak performance
- *Sleeping* is focused on recovery. This deep sleep state allows muscles to relax and repair, blood pressure to drop, and energy to be replaced
- *Nature* is about fresh air, UV exposure, and sensory experiences. The time and quality are down to the individual needs and circumstances
- *Tribe* means group support and accountability
- *Harmony* comes from inner strength and balance

Jane: That's a much fuller picture. And here's me thinking of exercise as a form of punishment.

Joyce: Ah, but I didn't say exercise; I said moving- anything from a stroll; to playing golf; to Zumba classes; and going for a run. It's different for every BODY. But it's the multi-benefits of endorphins which are the reward.

Jane: It's now becoming clear how those rewards improve self-esteem.

Joyce: The marker that is Self-esteem sits alongside a marker called Network (family, social, community, and digital), all points of contact. Striking the right balance here pushes you towards a positive, low-risk health space. The indicator being Connect (of the spirit), how well supported you are. Connect links to the next marker, Feelings, creating another domain called **SPIRIT**.

Jane: I can see why this domain is a spiritual space. I can't wait to hear what the rewards are.

Joyce: Yes, this domain is about the spirit within self and others. Here in this space, these rewards present differently:

- *Eating* is social and cultural, providing both comfort as well as celebration
- *Moving* is collective energy, ritualistic, and can create spiritual significance
- *Sleeping* is restorative. Like meditation, it lowers the heart rate and slows down breathing. A time to let go of distractions and runaway thoughts
- *Nature* represents an opportunity to spiritually link the physical to the non-physical, the concrete to the abstract
- *Tribe* represents a sense of belonging and community spirit
- *Harmony* is the freedom to be you and at one with the world

Jane: Wow! Joyce, you've just revealed another layer. I get it. The reward of sleep is different here, as are the rewards of eating and moving. I'm starting to see how they join up. I can see how the rewards propel you to positive outcomes in this domain.

Joyce: Again, it's no surprise. By taking care of our spiritual health, our emotions take care of themselves. Let's reveal the next domain. Alongside the Feelings marker sits the Thinking one. How we think determines how we behave and vice versa. Trauma, life events, and stressors can cloud thoughts. Equally, positive life events, good coping strategies, and resilience work to keep you safe. All of these can influence decision-making. These two measurable markers indicate Control (of the Mind).

Jane: Are we talking about stress management here? Or resilience?

Joyce: Both, actually. Coping strategies for the psychophysiological responses of your mind and body. Control as an indicator is your ability to predict emotional responses and understand behavioural patterns. When you join the Control indicator with the Health indicator, it opens up the domain of MIND.

Jane: So this is where mental health lives. I was hoping you wouldn't keep me waiting for the rewards on this one.

Joyce: Yes, this is where mental health meets physical health. Now that we've come full circle, let's look at the rewards for this domain:

- *Eating* is measured and mindful
- *Moving* is purposeful, a time to process and clear the head
- *Sleeping* is about duration and quality.* Seven to nine hours ideally, too little (insomnia), too much (Hypersomnia)
- *Nature* is about perspective and knowing when to change your space

- *Tribe* is about self-awareness and contributions– how to give and how to receive
- *Harmony* is stability and purpose

*Sleep quality is another measurable, which pulls together all aspects of sleep.

Jane: So the desired outcome must surely be peak mental performance?

Joyce: Not quite. Are you still viewing each of these domains in isolation? Imagine operating in the healthy zones in all three domains:

- MIND (Psychological)
- BODY (Physical)
- SPIRIT (Relationships, Social, Cultural)

These domains are interdependent; your mental, physical, and spiritual performance relies on their synergy. The power comes from understanding how each domain works and how individual outcomes impact each other. The final combined score symbolises your measure of success or not—the rewards in each domain matter. By chasing the rewards, you are equipping yourself with a healthier future.

Jane: How will you know when the rewards are working?

Joyce: Well, for one, your efforts are visually confirmed, and for two, you'll start to feel the difference. When your mental, physical, and spiritual health outcomes reach optimal levels for your age and body, you'll be content knowing you are doing your utmost *for yourself.*

Jane: What happens when you're in this optimal zone?

Joyce: You will know it, physically feel it and sense it. *You're walking tall*—the Warrior effect.

Jane: Thinking, Feeling, and Acting like a Warrior. Metaphorically speaking, of course.

Joyce: In each domain, for each of the simple six rewards, you will know if you're:

On Target – Green

Nearly there - Yellow

Falling short – Amber

Severely lacking - Red

Jane: Step by step, you've given me more insight and appreciation for what the holistic model means: Mind, Body, and Spirit. But more importantly, your position on the rewards indicators within each domain will promote an individual's measures of success—a far cry just from a single metric.

Joyce: I hope we finally recognise that the BMI is not the be-all and end-all with its inability to chart your efforts toward your *overall* goals.

Jane: It's the one measuring stick that feels less reward and more rebuke. It moves too slowly.

Joyce: You're right. This model gives you the domain priorities. Which domain is pulsing, and therefore which rewards are relevant? Where to focus and why.

Jane: You've done it, Joyce. Finally, a tool that *works with and for you.* By prompting you, charting your responses, and collating your data to give you a holistic picture.

Joyce: I wish I could take the credit for it. I've used it enough in my Wellness workshops. It's very popular. This model is known as **Risk2Reward®**.

Jane: What does this tool mean for the apples and pears of this world?

Joyce: Let's get stuck in and use it. We will use our known characters.

Jane: Quick recap for our listeners: Pear, as you will remember, was Red zoning (BMI high risk) for health, with a medical diagnosis (depression) and prescription for anti-depressants. Meanwhile, Apple was Yellow zoning (BMI low risk) for health but was also medically diagnosed (hypertension) and flagged as potentially high risk for stroke. So that's where we left them at the end of **Risk2Reward®**, and that's how they arrived here.

Joyce: So what's going on? *Firstly a nod to the professionals and their involvement. As a wellness expert, I will always defer to their knowledge and expertise. All our clients are referred to our centre as part of an adjunctive treatment plan.* To begin with, let's imagine these avatars have completed their self-efficacy inputs and have scored accordingly. With the algorithms in place, they have each placed to a greater or lesser extent on each indicator which points to an overall positioning within each domain. We begin with Pear.

Jane: How is she presenting in the Mind, Body, and Spirit domains?

Joyce: Let's start with what we know. Her BMI has put her into the high-risk Health indicator. However, the scores in this Risk2Reward model point towards the high-risk zones in all domains, with the Body domain pulsing the most.

Jane: We've already established that she's lonely and depressed. She's eating poorly, and she's not moving very much. So if her loneliness is due to being cut off or feeling cut off from everyone, she can remedy that, but maybe less so in the Pandemic.

Joyce: If she can't, being unable to or has no agency, then others need to step in. Studies show that loneliness comes with a health warning. Raised stress levels and sleep problems, both affect physical and mental health.

Jane: Correct. Loneliness is a state of mind. Isolation is measurable. And, indeed, some people cope better with it. Think of the happy hermits. While others feel tortured by solitary confinement, the hermits may thrive.

Joyce: Exactly.

Jane: How should she reward herself?

Joyce: Let's be realistic. First, let's acknowledge that Covid was an exceptional time. Life events played a role too. Even so, not all Pears would have found themselves positioned like her. This Pear is especially reactive. Life events happen, and her emotional responses coupled with her behaviours toward them, have always played out in the extreme. She's primed to react to these triggers in a certain way. There is a high probability that she will be allostatically loaded. From the time she was in play, she's accumulated stress after stress. Inflammation and compromised immunity underpin all the behavioural hazards in her life's journey.

Jane: Now that she is in the healthcare zone for mental health, she will have access to professionals and treatments. They will guide her well.

Joyce: At our wellness centre, we will run in parallel with the professionals. We'd be urging her to focus on the following rewards: healthy eating, moving for her heart health, sleeping to recover, getting out into fresh air, and ensuring she's UV exposed and thus experiencing the nature reward. Her turnaround starts with incremental steps. Harmony will follow once she can balance her energy. Changing direction will have her start to collect the simple rewards. Control, Health, and Connect in balance may eventually be within her reach.

Jane: By using the Body as a starting point, the Mind tends to follow, and that's the bonus of active self-care. This route is well known.

Joyce: Their knock-on effect brings holistic balance. Let's look at what motivates her.

Jane: She could think she still has a third of her life left.

Joyce: Statistically speaking, yes. But her focus would now be living the remainder of her life in good health.

Jane: What about the Spirit domain?

Joyce: Perhaps she feels cut off with Covid and the lockdowns. Who knows what her network of family, friends, and community comprises? Like everyone in the pandemic, she may be limited to her digital network.

Jane: Let's move on. What about Apple?

Joyce: From Apple's self-efficacy scoring, she is positioned in the low-risk zone for the Body and Spirit domains. The domain Mind represents a definite wobble—no surprise when you think about what was in play for her.

Jane: Let's have another look at that last play. The self, plus any unrest in her local environment, against the backdrop of world events, can potentially jeopardise her. There are three personal jeopardies in play: age, female, and ethnicity.

Joyce: Generally, an ageing ethnic female may feel emotionally vulnerable if she's a minority and marginalised. These jeopardies can derail anyone, given the circumstances.

Jane: We covered this before in the game of Risk. These are recognisable stressors.

Joyce: How is her mental state affected? What do we know so far?

Jane: Her last Risk play has shown a change in her risk level. Her energy balance is out of whack. Fear is a trigger for emotional stress. It plays out in her body. Perhaps her troubled mind has affected her sleep. Restrictions and lockdowns would have compromised her social and natural rhythms.

Joyce: Even the best of us, doing all the right things, can still be thrown off course when a calamity card is played. As a key worker in the trenches, it's no surprise that PTSD is a hazard in play too.

Jane: She has navigated herself and her risk levels quite successfully thus far. She's done well.

Joyce: As careful as she is, the post-pandemic emotional burden will feel different. The triggers will be different. That's what accumulative stress does. Allostatic stress does not dissipate that quickly, if at all. Weathering takes its toll.

Jane: So what should her focus be now?

Joyce: Recognising that post-pandemic is an opportunity to reassess, to chart the way forward.

Jane: So, what is a good starting point for her?

Joyce: Apple is one of many women like this. They are self-aware and keep themselves in check using available tools and methods.

Jane: Are you saying that she will self-correct?

Joyce: Very likely, based on her play so far. It's all about finding your route and creating the balance you need.

Jane: … and that's her harmony… until menopause.

Joyce: There is a reason we haven't got to that yet.

Jane: Saving the best for last, hey?

Joyce: Before we overlay the menopause, let's appreciate what **Risk2Reward®** does. It encompasses all the variables. Women come in all shapes and sizes. We are genetically different. We have various cultural influences with differing socio-economic means. And we may have a variety of disabilities, hidden or otherwise.

Jane: Not to mention your identity and your societal fit.

Joyce: Let's assess one of the women in my clinic. She may surprise you. She's a professional, holds a responsible job, and is trusted and admired by many. At first glance, she's BMI-perfect, enviably fit, and strong.

Jane: I hate her already, ha ha.

Joyce: You won't hate her when you hear she came to me pre-pandemic and disclosed that she felt broken and emotionally vulnerable. Her scores on the **Risk2Reward**® model confirmed that she needed to focus on her Spirit domain. All was not lost.

Jane: So if she was pulsing in the Spirit domain. Without knowing the details, what was her route to self-healing? Assuming she has self-balanced.

Joyce: For a start, the **Risk2Reward**® tool helped her explore any emotional burdens unreleased from her childhood, including any other lingering demons in her more recent history, current dilemmas, and their related stressors. Her Connect score was also low. This woman, let's refer to her as Celery, revealed a fourth jeopardy.

Jane: A fourth? I'm intrigued.

Joyce: Yes. She is ageing, she's female, she's a woman of colour, and she's a member of the LGBTQ+ community.

Jane: Quite a smorgasbord of revelations.

Joyce: That's the power of this tool. It's her inputs, her choices, and her responses that have revealed this outcome. From that, she was able to set a course for chasing the right sort of rewards to satisfy the Spirit domain.

Jane: So she changed direction.

Joyce: Yes. From food as fuel to seeing it as social, comfort, or celebration. From movement as fitness to now ritualistic, with spiritual significance. Sleep, rather than just recovery, like meditation, is now restorative. Nature is not only about UV exposure. It now also presents an opportunity to link the physical and non-physical.

Jane: Are we talking tree-hugging?

Joyce: Why not? Forest bathing is a known de-stressor. Originating in Japan, now practised far and wide. So the next reward - tribe is an interesting one for her.

Jane: How so?

Joyce: For her, tribe has always represented accountability. Now, it represents a sense of belonging, recognising her community. So her harmony will come from her freedom to just be herself.

Jane: I get it. At one with the world.

Joyce: Another way of changing her paradigm is thinking of her emotional vulnerability as her skill.

Jane: Explain, please. Why is that a skill?

Joyce: Rather than continuing to mask difficult emotions, she must acknowledge these first and see their power rather than their weakness.

Jane: Sadness, shame, uncertainty, fear, etc., is within us all. How do we turn a perceived weakness into a strength? Is it when we learn to love our authentic selves?

Joyce: Well, take vulnerability, and let's reframe it. Rather than rejection or failure, consider it at the heart of building meaningful experiences. Hard as it may be, exposing our true selves and being authentic builds empathy with others. We share feelings that others can reciprocate.

Jane: Exactly. As society evolves and becomes more liberated, it smooths out the jeopardies towards acceptance.

Joyce: With gratitude following. Let me explain. By acknowledging the goodness in self and life, you connect with something more significant. It's all about the connection, whether it be other people, nature, or a higher power.

Jane: Celery must allow vulnerability and gratitude to be her greatest strengths.

Joyce: Absolutely. And a lesson to us all. None of us dare judge.

Now that we've explored what's at the core of each character let's overlay this with Menopause.

Jane: Finally. I knew we'd get there in the end. Does menopause skew the picture?

Joyce: Well, it all depends on each individual's narrative. We know that in the same way every woman is unique, so too is their menopausal journey. That's what this Model demonstrates.

Jane: My listeners already know about measuring symptoms' frequency and intensity.

Joyce: So rather than think of menopause and its symptoms as running alongside core health, it's integrated with an ageing body with its health history and genetic blueprint. It touches on all the domains causing different stress levels at other times.

Jane: I see how these narratives of menopause play out in my friends. Some are suffering. Others celebrate newfound freedom from a lack of periods and pain. And some shrug it off and get on with life in much the same way as before.

Joyce: You've correctly identified the three well-known narratives of menopause across all its stages:

- Distressed
- Metamorphic
- Normal

Jane: Let's remember we've also got life events chiming in at different times.

Joyce: Indeed. Midlife is multi-layered and complex. This tool is there to check in, assess and rebalance periodically—a road map to good health for the next three decades.

Now is the time to equip yourself to become a warrior for the next stage of life.

Jane: As women, our strength is in numbers. And we know that numbers drive change. So now is the time we support each other rather than compete.

So when they shout, "Stay healthy," we can ROAR back with certainty, "We will!"

Joyce: Well said, Jane.

Jane: Thank you, Joyce, my friend, for your insights and valuable contribution. It's been a pleasure having you in the studio with me.

And to my listeners, the last two segments have been quite deep and deedy.

So tune in next time for a bit of fun and games.

| 11 |

Erica's story

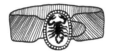

"I'll be damned if I have to wear this one notch out." I said aloud. Sucking in my tummy with all my might, I tried again to get the pin into the notch, failed, and then shouted, "Bugger!"

My family called up the stairs, "You all right?"

"Yes, fine," I lied irritatingly while thinking obsessively about the recent struggle. Every notch out represents a stone gained, even if the scales didn't agree.

This is not just any belt; this is my favourite belt, my miracle. It gives me that wasp-like waist, the cinched look when done up. It's become increasingly uncomfortable lately, so if I can still get it on and done up, wearing it will silence the critics. Visually it will make a statement, recover the situation with Ollie, and resume play.

The belt in question is a Prada belt on sale in the outlet shop in Italy - so effectively a double bargain. I bought it years ago. I felt at the time somewhat disappointed that my Italian grandparents barely registered my precious find (they don't 'do' labels; they are far too humble), but they did appreciate that it gave me joy and that it was exquisite Italian leather.

For me, that belt represented many things. No longer the needy young woman, carrying an extra three stone in weight and the stigma of being from a different class. It symbolised constriction and armour juxtaposed with liberation too. The notch on the belt was always my gauge of being in control. And being in control was cocking a snook at the critics from my past.

Four years after my doctorate, I'd come from being swamped as a mature PhD student whilst juggling motherhood and enduring the subsequent drudge of working for a charity and publishing paper after paper. Then to emergence. I became the person to inspire others, challenge them, and impart knowledge rather than absorb it. That Prada belt also represented transformation. It was the holiday treat that celebrated my new job as a lecturer at the local university. I needed it to feel groomed in this new arena. That was years ago.

The belt is now a staple piece of my wardrobe, an old friend, and it, like me, is well maintained and has worn well.

Ollie is my favourite student; super bright and cheeky. He hasn't written me off. I look forward to our banter, but recently we'd had a clumsy exchange,

"No, Ollie, your reply makes you sound thick," I duelled.

He retorted, "What, as thick as your waistline?"

Ouch!

My face must have shown the group that I was stung and un-characteristically back footed because not one student had tittered. Ollie knew that he had misfired; he had stepped over the mark. Things had turned awkward with no recovery. In my head, I asked myself, was I oversensitive? He couldn't have meant it because the black belt does give my silhouette the illusion of a waist. I feel supported and strong whenever I wear it, especially when standing in front of young eyes that constantly judge me. Aware that my sharp intelligence and wit have always made me a little prickly. I am a force to be reckoned with, or at least that's what people say. I am used to not being hugely popular, but I take comfort in that at least my polished image is impressive and, to most, appealing. I trade on it; it gives me power and has a currency of its own.

And, I don't need to be liked by everyone, only those I value. I have an ego, for sure. Twas always the case. On the one hand, always secure in my thinking. (I had form: head girl at school and president of the debating society at university).

On the other hand, less secure in the metamorphosis of my changing body. I was always clean, brushed, perfumed, and never without vermillion lipstick. A painful jilt and the weight loss it sparked crafted this trademark look. I like what I invented. Never will I feel that vulnerable again. I know the red lipstick shows off my Irish green eyes that sparkle when I smile; thank you, Dad. They turn Pernod yellowy green when I'm hot-tempered and frowning; thank you, Mum. My family tells me I have made babies cry when I arch my brow. An exaggeration, but I can play up to my caricature if required. Maybe I revel too much in my reputation, but my students are mostly admiring, and with my candour, they all trust me. Everyone knows where they stand. I know I'm competent, and my intentions towards my students are honourable until they take liberties.

I wish I could say the same about the university staff. The admin staff are ok; it's just with the rest of the academic team where I have a few issues. My colleagues find me 'difficult' – Good!

Academic meetings can be very political and dominated by too many fragile egos trying to force their agendas. As a result, any progress is painfully slow. Too often, meetings can turn into meetings about meetings that go nowhere. Unfortunately for them, I call out any disingenuous remarks. Maybe I was being too combative with my reply to the head of the faculty. "Greg, I'd like to agree with you, but that would make us both wrong."

It was appreciated by most but lost on him. Hey ho. He *is* a bit of an arse, and anyway, I'm well-published, so he has to put up with me.

Just lately, I've waited too long to get my point across, and I've forgotten what I was going to say – maddening. Anger keeps me focused but doesn't give the right impression, as my colleagues always think I'm spoiling for a fight. Is this what they mean about brain fog? If I feel that I'm losing my credibility in the faculty meetings, is it only a matter of time before I lose it publicly? I've gone from being mildly irritated to, on occasion, fearful. I've never been afraid of public speaking in my life! I don't recognise myself lately. The feeling is so random, so unpredictable. Is it early-onset dementia? Always a cruel disease, and the irony is not lost on me.

Now the heat waves are coming. I know patience isn't my thing, and others are usually aware that trouble is brewing when I say, "What's the purpose of this discussion?" Or "Can we cut to the chase?" Even when I give a deep sigh, that alone can ruffle feathers. I don't care. But now I have to leave the room. When a heatwave begins to creep above my silk neckerchief, my latest tactic is to excuse myself and go to the loo. I don't have any bladder issues, but the cubicle gives me space to recover.

Recently my yanking of the paper towel in the ladies' loo drew the attention of a colleague.

"What did that towel ever do to you?" She asked as she watched me violently drying my hands. "The meeting, as usual, is a waste of time," I replied. "Trust me; I'm on best behaviour. But it doesn't stop me from fantasising about wringing somebody's neck!" We both laughed as we recognised the likely recipient.

She said, "You're the same as ever, Erica. The pandemic didn't affect you."

"I suppose so," I replied. "But like everyone, we muddled along, grappling with Zoom. Made even more challenging with my daughter turning vegan."

"How old is Savannah now?"

"Seventeen going on 22!"

"It must be fun with you and your mini-me in your household."

"Not sure about fun, but always interesting. Oh, and my father had a stroke."

I wasn't about to disclose how alarmed I was when my Father had that stroke and how pitiful it was to see this once erudite man struggle with his slurred speech. It was cruel for him and for us to witness. Nor did I let on how deeply affected I was by my son Will, deciding to move in with his girlfriend during the lockdown.

"Anyway, must get back. Once more into the breach."

I pick up my discarded scarf and put it back in my bag. Never mind the hand towel; I hoped that my colleagues hadn't thought to strangle *me* with my scarf!

My hot flushes were full throttle. They were so unexpected, with no apparent rhyme or reason. My periods were all over the place too. I'd gone a couple of months without any then, surprise! Whoosh, right in the middle of a lecture. Thank goodness I wasn't wearing white and I was standing. I acted out that I was having a coughing fit so I could excuse myself. I panicked in the loos when I realised I had only one tampon and a slim sanitary towel. I layered my pants so full of toilet tissue that I'm sure I walked back to the lecture hall, legs astride, like a sumo wrestler. After that episode, I swapped bags and made sure that I always carried a whole pack of STs. Another couple of months went by with nothing and no sign of a visit from the decorators or 'Aunt Flo'. Then they were back, periods as regular as clockwork again, along with my customary craving for salami. It was all so bewildering. I thought, what other contingency plans do I need? I'm always in the damned loo!

My kids had noticed a change in me too. Will said I was losing my touch. They had swapped updates about the scorpion within me misfiring. Obviously, 'scorpion' was code for me when I had my time of the month. I was unaware that I was grumpy, but when Savannah started her periods, Will had warned her that she could expect "to lash out randomly, like Mum. Dad and I know when to take off," he'd said. Savannah wasn't so lucky; she remained in my firing line and took a different tack. She confided in me about my label. From then on, 'The Scorpion' was mother and daughter code for an apology because of unnecessarily cruel comments. With irregular periods, they are unsure if and when the scorpion will resurface. Perhaps I'll grow into a benign, gentle old lady. As if!

At work, it's lunchtime. The canteen has a routine, and so do I. It represents another obstacle course to navigate. Must eat? Should eat? Could eat? A fellow diner appears to be meticulously sorting out the sequence of her plate. Our eyes meet, and I wonder if she has the same tipping point from enjoyment to cut-off as I do. Maybe not; her spark has gone. I play safe; I know the rules.

After lunch, I try on the sacred black belt again. This time, I got it to the final notch by stretching it to its limit. I caught myself exclaiming, "Did it!!" Then, feeling triumphant, albeit more than uncomfortable, I reassured myself that my blood supply should remain for the entire lecture if I remained standing and avoided bending down. Privately I congratulated myself and thought, *Yes, the wasp's waist is back, on guard, dear Ollie!*

Seeing Ollie come down the corridor, stopping dead in his tracks. The look in his eyes told me that I was back to looking fit and dangerous.

Swiftly recovering, Ollie says, "Hi Erica, I was going to ask for an extension for the assignment. I have a family crisis, and my Dad needs me."

"Ollie, as you know, my usual response to that request is, Never; all deadlines for assignments are absolute; they should be delivered immediately if not sooner."

I studied his face and saw it appear drained of colour. "But Ollie, I'm not a monster; I can see that you're troubled; you're practically the colour of celadon."

He looked confused.

"Look it up," I said. "Ok, let's be realistic; when can you get it to me?"

"Friday?" he offered.

"No, next Tuesday it is!" I replied. "On two conditions: One, you include the term Celadon in your submission; two, you don't tell anyone that I've gone soft."

Ollie gave a faint smile, "Thank you, Erica."

Such a lovely lad, I thought. His parents must be so proud. He's exactly the type I would wish for Savannah.

After my lecture, I felt pleased that things were back to almost normal, or they would be as soon as I got out of this instrument of torture. But, feeling rueful, I'm just not ready to concede, permanently discard and mourn my favourite black belt. There must be another way, another yardstick demonstrating that I measure up, to silence my haunting critics.

There was a time when I *was* judged, and it hurt—judged for not having the required greyhound figure. My first love, our first naked encounter, him measuring me up, fingers like callipers, and his crude assessment of my waist and hips. "You're very upholstered, aren't you? Built more for comfort, not speed."

At home, Ed's relieved that I'm back. He and Savannah had a heated discussion earlier, and it's rattled him. There's certainly an atmosphere that is palpable and lingering. It's been a long time since I've seen him this angry. Moving house with the incompetent solicitors was memorable – I thought he would combust until I had to step in. But our biggest row was when I spent my legacy from Uncle Stefano and pushed to do my doctorate when we still had young children. He accused me of being selfish, a bad mother, but I successfully argued that I deserved a career too. Being a full-time mother was slowly, or not so slowly, turning me insane. "I'm miserable, Ed. I'm envious of you every time you escape to work." I added that neither of us likes housework, so it would be better to have paid help if we can afford it. I was right; having help paid off. Overall my decision preserved both our sanity and our careers. All our home helpers have added richness to the kids' lives. Weekends were, and still are, for family and, thus, sacred.

But now, I'm curious. It's unusual; Ed is usually the peacemaker between mother and daughter. So what on earth went on to upset him? He's generally putty in our darling daughter's hands.

Ed exclaims, "According to Savannah, everything I suggested in the fridge was inappropriate; not enough plant-based choices. Apparently, I'm an out-of-touch dinosaur; she's becoming an incredibly angry young woman. I blame that, Greta,"

I stifle a smile. I also think Savannah is too impassioned at the moment. Probably for all the right reasons, but she's losing the argument if she can alienate her even-tempered and ridiculously soft dad.

"She's seventeen, Ed. Her hormones are raging, and she's found her cause, just like we did in our day. Better that she voices her thoughts and concerns rather than go silent and muted, don't you think?"

"You two are more alike and can ebb and flow more easily. Would you deal with her, please?" He pleaded. "Of course. You won't believe me if I tell you that I plan to. Softly, softly ...," I whispered. "Ha, no, I don't believe you but good luck!" he chuckled.

Swiftly changing the subject, I ask, "When will the golf club be open again?"

Ed: "As soon as the green keepers say so as there are changes in the green structure that needs to settle and ..."

I'm too tired and too hungry to listen or care truly.

"Dinner will be ready soon." Must remember to log all the cherry tomatoes I ate in the car on the way home. I hope no one misses them.

"Ed, let's eat – Savannah can help herself to beans on toast when she's calmed down."

The next day, we both worked from home: me, marking and lesson planning; Ed- re-designing an engineering problem. It was a calm and productive day spent at our laptops. So after work, we took our electric bikes out, and after a long ride, we agreed that we both felt better for the exercise. Life felt good, and we were grateful for connecting with the natural world. Except, I felt a little lightheaded for the journey back. Ed was worried and commented about me having just soup for lunch and declining to eat the bread rolls. "Not the smartest idea, Erica". He frogmarched me into the village shop and bought two bananas. Outside, I lasciviously ate one of them. Ed matched me audibly, exclaiming "yum" with every bite, making the scene increasingly sexual. That is until a stranger stepped out of the shop, and both immediately went silent like naughty school kids.

I remember thinking gratefully, *I struck gold when I found Ed.*

Later in the kitchen, at the bin, scraping away most of my dinner, Ed walks in ...uh, oh.

"Darling, we're not in Africa, you know. So are you starving yourself again?"

Africa was a lifetime ago—my gap year. After the heartache of that first love, I had re-invented myself to be that greyhound. Then, built for speed and not comfort and brandishing a top honours degree, I met Ed. And when he told me, "I find a woman with intelligence behind the eyes, very sexy," I succumbed. We fell in love.

"You got very ill then, and it scared you; now you're scaring me!"

I was never out of control. Even then, I could stay safe, never crossing the line.

"Savanna's worried too; you're getting thin and obsessing again," Ed trailed off.

My whole raison d'être has been about control. Lately, I have felt like the wheels are falling off. Let me do a checklist. One, I'm peri-menopausal, and the flushes and fogs are getting in the way. Two, my daughter is rebelling with shockwaves across our home. Three, I'm fading in front of the youthful gaze in the lecture theatre. Four, I'm haunted by the visions of my beloved Father, and he's not even dead yet. To top it all: my belt says I'm no longer measuring up. And if another person tells me to put things into perspective, I will have to poison them.

Back to reality.

"I'm losing the plot, Ed. I feel like I'm waning. In more ways than one."

"You look the same to me. I fell in love with you back then, and I'm still in love with you now. So you're undeniably a one-off. Pain in the arse then, a pain in the arse now, but I wouldn't have it any other way."

"Then don't rebuke me! I'm not too thin. I can't do my damn favourite belt up! And I blame you for providing temptations from your wine cellar."

"Yup, I just knew it would be my fault – but darling, you drank more red wine than me," he laughs, rolling his eyes.

Not letting it go, he said, "I think I was savouring each sip whilst you kept toasting to 'antioxidants' and draining each glass."

I really couldn't remember.

"Anyway, what if your belt eases a bit, we're all going to face the middle-aged spread; it happens to us all," he sighed.

"Wash your mouth out, Edward! That is not going to happen, not on my watch!"

Time to power down.

"Ready for bed, darling?" Asks Ed. "I've got the paper here for us to finish the cryptic crossword."

My rituals began.

I started to unpack my day with every layer that I discarded.

Hanging the jacket up that helped me triumph with the Dean.

Shedding the sleeveless silk shirt that showed off my sculpted arms (the envy of all my female students), thank you, trainer Zac.

Stepping out of my Ferragamo's, I've definitely earned my well-heeled status.

Removing my matching and expensive underwear not needed to satisfy Ed, but absolutely needed to satisfy ME.

Then I set about removing all traces of the mask from my face—a four-step approach: Strip, tone, nourish, seal.

And all this before the final ablutions.

Groomed to the nth degree: Manicure intact, check. Pedicure intact, check. Hairless where it matters, laser appointment in the diary, check. Skin nourished, now supple, check. I am as naked and as exposed as I dare to be. I slip into bed.

"Darling, what is 'Mythical phoenix and its European resurge?' Two words. The second word, eleven letters."

"Easy, The Renaissance."

"That's my Erica. Knew you'd get it."

A week on.

We've had a good week until Savannah insisted we watch 'The Game Changers' on Sunday, followed by 'Cowspiracy.' We should never have agreed to watch both in one day. The mood was grim. As a family, we discussed intelligently and decided that both films were very well done and informative but chilling. Ed and I agreed, and I was proud of Savannah for her excellent values. She's strident and unafraid to speak up for what she genuinely believes in. However, the whole Sunday afternoon was very intense and exhausting. We all decided to forego our Sunday walk –a big mistake. Things went from bad to worse, with Savannah piling everything she disapproved of on the kitchen table. It was a step too far. The cost: pounds and pounds of food, leather accessories, and cosmetics, all to be thrown out? NO! I felt that our house had been ransacked, and we felt abused. She wanted to change the world at record-breaking speed and to change *our* world at home in a blink of an eye. It was too much. All three of us got very irate, and none truly listened, only to say, "Good point, but…" It was an ugly end to a day that was supposed to be about rest.

I do know my daughter, though. She'll not rest. I decided to sleep on it and choose my moment to have a planned discussion rather than a debate. I sensed that Ed felt awkward in his own home and probably fearful about his folks coming to visit at the end of the month. I only hoped they'd bring jam, not honey, and no dairy products from their farm. Maybe Ed would give a diplomatic heads-up warning. Hmm, we both pondered in bed; clever boxing required.

The next day Savannah was still snarking, "Dad's still in a foul mood, I see."

"I'm calling it now, Savannah. SCORPION, you're it!" I reply. "Put your tail down. He agrees more than he disagrees with you. He eats little meat in the scheme of things, and for a man his age with his background, give him a break."

"Yeah, whatever," she says, "So he's of farming stock. Time to think of the carbon footprint."

"C'mon, our diet is mostly Mediterranean. We keep adjusting. We're all learning. We've moved increasingly to a more plant-based and whole grain diet. So give *us* a break"

"Not really, Mum. You have your salami fix at your time of the month – which is disgusting by the way. Processed and fatty, what are you doing? You're a hypocrite!"

She's right. Even I don't know what that's all about. I have an inexplicable craving, always have had. "I don't eat much of it, just a couple of slices."

I have no idea why I crave salami on the first day of my period, but I can't remember ever not eating it. I continued, "You, however, Miss, get through tons of expensive dark chocolate at that, whether vegan or not. I know because I'm paying for it!"

"I'll bloody pay for it myself! At least it'll be vegan." Shouted Savannah. "Our whole family could so easily go that way. So why not?"

"Hold on, not so fast; there is still much to learn and get used to."

Ed and I are more open to these changes than most and, indeed, applaud this movement, but we know that we need to tread more carefully and respectfully with the older generation.

"You'll offend your grandparents if you strongly criticize their choices, old habits die hard."

"I disagree, a softly softly approach sucks. Don't you get it? There's no time, our planet is in chaos, and change is urgent."

"Savannah, it's a much bigger deal. Very complex. None of us truly know what it will take to feed the world. So please take care."

This passionate daughter of ours does indeed need to take care. To play it smart because if she continues to bang the drum too loudly, she may turn people deaf to her message. No one wants to be offended and shamed for their choices. It needs more tolerance and understanding both ways. She'll have to find out the hard way. And once again, Ed and I will be here to pick up the pieces.

"You can talk, Mum. If everyone ate like you, we wouldn't be here. There'd be a bloody surplus!"

Perché?

"Mum, you keep challenging me on my vital AAs and B12, but you don't eat anything! Black coffee and carrot sticks don't cut a good diet, do they?"

"I've lost my appetite; lately, that's all," I said. "You don't know what I eat during the working day, so that's enough!"

"Yes, it is, Mum; it's enough that you don't eat enough! You eat all the right things, just not enough of those things. Dad and I are worried. You've got all the books - you wax lyrically about your nutrition gurus, quoting chapter and verse, but don't follow the guidelines yourself."

"Respect, Savannah!"

"Don't pull rank on me now, Mum! And you know that Dad spends too much time at the golf club talking to a curvy blond? She's a nutritionist."

"That's a low blow, Savannah. SCORPION!"

We parted as adversaries. Ridiculous considering we agreed more than we disagreed. It turns out that growth is painful in all generations.

Note to self; *I will meet Ed at the golf club bar for a surprise drink. Sizing up the competition and conspicuously eating lots of nuts.*

What was I thinking? I turned up unannounced at the club—no curvy nutritionist in sight. There *was* no opposition. Ed was not at the bar. Instead, he was at the restaurant tucking into a plate with a two-inch steak and chips.

"Ed, that's the size of half a cow. Shame on you!"

Looking suitably chastised and ashamed, he said, "Erica, I have to have my meat fix, and this is where I partake."

"That, my dear, is a two-stroke penalty. **Fore** one, you're eating meat, and two, that pun was woeful. So I'll leave you to **chip** and **slice** your way through that lot while I go and get a drink."

I walked away smugly and left him chuckling as I thought, *no competition.*

Later, I watched Savannah making amends, currying favour with her Father. Unintentionally her movements and her vocal tone mimic a seductive lure. I recognise that she's transitioning, too, from a girl to a woman. Her lithe body is effortlessly lean, a machine very different from mine. She's free from doubts and in-securities, mostly courtesy of Ed's genes. As well as a loving and entitled environment that Ed and I have worked hard to provide. This freedom, her sexual awakening, and her power of growing enchantments are yet another reminder of my bloom diminishing. I refuse to be that clichéd dowdy bird resenting plumage. I *will* retain my currency and rejoice in my daughter's coming of age.

Now for my adjustments and re-invention. This phoenix will rise again.

Time to power up.

Stepping from the shower. Deodorant on, check. Body lotion - scented and supple, check. Teeth, flossed, brushed, mouth washed, check. Face, double cleansed, toned, serum one, serum two, eye cream, moisturise, and tinted SPF. Check. At a significant cost, the canvas is prepped.

Now to recreate the mask.

Step one – conceal: dark eye circles, age spots, blemishes.

Step two – blur: lip lines, elevenses, crow's feet.

Step three – contour: hairline, temple, cheekbones, jaw.

Step four – blend all and seal.

Step five – fill, brush, seal: brows.

Step six – curl: eyelashes.

Step seven – define: the upper lid - eyelash line, lower lid – eyelash line, tapering out from the centre. And blend.

Step eight – shadow: base colour to the lid, darker shade to the crease, highlight brow bones. And blend.

Step nine - layer: mascara. One coat, then two.

Step ten – blush: cheekbones from the mid-eye out. (Think Mohican war paint) And blend.

Step eleven - outline: lips, and colour in. (Remember finger pop to remove excess product)

Step twelve – perfume: pulse points. (neck: left, right, and wrists)

Mask complete. Now smile. Or is it brace? As here came the in-laws.

I'd already asked Savannah to make the vegan chilli again. It was utterly delicious last time; even Ed complimented it. I wondered if she thought it a clever idea to make it for the in-laws. After all, proof would be in the eating. "Do I have to stay for this, Mum?" She asked. "If I go, I can avoid arguments and Dad would be more comfortable."

"I appreciate the sentiment on this occasion," I said. "But you can't keep exiting tricky situations to keep the peace. They are good people, Savannah. Meat growing, meat-eating, farming people. Not evil. As farmers go, they are responsible and great with their herds and flocks. They truly value their stock. Their perspective may be different from yours. So please don't berate them."

"My challenge for you is to ensure this dish is so delicious that even they would have to concede that there's a credible alternative to meat. Change is possible. I'll leave it with you."

I then went up to the bedroom, and there was a new belt with a note on my side of the bed.

This is pleather, Mum. BTW – don't worry, you'll always look great,
Love you,
Savannah
Xx

It was indeed a good-looking belt. I tried it on. I attached my vintage scorpion clasp, looked in the mirror, and admired my cinched-in waist.

I called down the stairs.

"Thank you, Savannah, I love it!! And … I love you! Onwards!"

There is always a way.

| 12 |

The Vanity (Warrior) Project

As Jane Austen said:

"Vanity and pride are different, though the words are often used synonymously. A person may be proud without being vain. Pride relates more to our opinion of ourselves, vanity to what we would have others think of us."

Is it pride or vanity that keeps the hag at bay? It begs the question. Who is judging whom?

Years on, we are reflecting on the archaic beauty standards imposed upon us by the patriarchal culture of the day. Over centuries, that definition of beauty keeps changing back and forth until…

Here we are, in the present day, the digital age, where bodies are still youthful and slender, teeth are perfect, butts and breasts are more than a handful, lips are plump, brows and lashes are dark and feathery, hair is extended, skins are flawlessly perfect and tanned. All this flaunted to a mass audience. Social media or otherwise.

Beauty standards are superficial and forever chasing youth. Look at the representation of the older woman as a role model. With silver hair and a few wrinkles (as a nod to midlife), they are depicted as having glowing skin, slim bodies, perfect teeth, and always bloody smiling. A standard that may only be attainable by a few. Whether you're born with it, buying it, peddling it, or chasing it, the question remains. Who designed the blueprint for midlife beauty?

So who should make the rules now? Who fights for change, recognising the diversity around the globe of women's body shapes past, present, and future. The answer is WE SHOULD! We want to celebrate our changing bodies: from puberty to motherhood and finally in and beyond menopause. Following on from earlier battles for emancipation, education, and reproductive rights, we all agree; now is the time to re-write the script for the beauty industry.

Think about what you will need to face the world. Will you need your mask of protection or the mask of power? Either dialling down to bare minimum comfort or dialling up to battle-ready confidence in preparation for harsh scrutiny. So where is the authentic you? It starts from within—your pride. Vitality and confidence always shine louder than any lipstick.

This metaphorical story is about six fiery queens from different realms in various stages of midlife and menopause. Having found their happily ever after, these fair maidens of olde have now aged. They now confront the mirrors and sense their magic has gone. What will make these queens from the Kingdoms of olde, become the Warrior Queens of the present and the future?

Over twenty-one days, they are marooned on an island with a weekly challenge. They have to perform individually and as a group, with two degrees of exposure: self-acknowledgement and recognition within the group. The only magic rests with the island's mystical guide.

Their story begins here:

Queens arrive separately by boat. They were assigned staggered arrival times and, upon landing at the dock, were led in all their splendour and finery (and all their travel bags) to their tiny cabin in amongst the palm trees. Each studio cabin has a bed and a small vanity for their belongings. A modest en suite reveals a bright copper framed mirror on the wall. But it's no good as the glass is opaque and obscures their image. Never mind, they've each brought their compact mirrors. They soon realise they are hopelessly overdressed and weighed down with baggage. There's not much room to swing a ... cape.

Bee, relieved at having made it to the loo on time, thinks, Phew, nearly had a wee moment there. Then as she powders her nose using her tiny compact, she wonders, Why give us a mirror if it's no bloody good. Gosh, I look my age today. I bet I'm the oldest one here.

They've all arrived, and although they can hear the mutters and the moans of their extremely dissatisfied neighbours, they know to wait until the gong sounds before meeting in the communal area. They use this time to freshen up. Thank goodness for all the lotions and potions they've brought. At least they will face their peers with their masks firmly in place.

One cabin inhabitant mutters, "I'm grubby and need a shower. Otherwise, I won't be Ping, but Pong. Wonder if I can squeeze in some training before dinner?"

All the instructions are preceded by a GONG and delivered by tannoy.

One by one, they leave their cabins and make their way to the meeting hut.

GONG: "Welcome, Queens. Your refreshments await. Use this time to introduce yourselves before the games commence."

Two queens simultaneously turn and face the group. Neither wants to back down.

"Hi," they both begin. There's polite laughter in the group before one finally gestures to the other to go ahead.

"I'm Kink. But that's for me to know why and for you all to find out, eventually. It may be everything or nothing to do with my hair."

"The name's Queen Grimhilde, but call me Barb, not Grim. You may have heard about me. And know that seven is not my favourite number."

With a shy wave, a voice pipes up, "Just call me T, short for Tiana. Are there frogs here? Ugh, I can't stand frogs."

"The name is Ping. Honestly, not sure why I'm here. Not into beauty parades. Where are all the men?"

"Hello, my lovelies. To Bee or not to Bee, that's not the question. It's just my name."

"Greetings. My name is Ella. I've recently been through the mill and back. My cautionary tale where magic is involved is, be careful what you wish for."

The queens continue to size each other up. A few wear their finery with confidence and authority, while others are swamped, restricted, and liberally using their fans. Some look bored, some look cross, and others look alarmed. All were thinking, What's this all about?

GONG: "Queens, you're all overdressed for the games ahead. It's time to get real and level up. **Time to go RAW !**"

POOF. All their finery disappears, and they find themselves in white shorts, white tee-shirts and robust trainers, with all traces of makeup removed.

"Level up? Level up! More like level down if you ask me," says Barb, looking down at her sturdy unbranded trainers.

GONG: "Queens, whether you believe in freeing the nip or needing support, the relevant engineering is available in your cabin."

The queens look around the group before five of the six gracefully turn and walk with increasing speed to their cabins—some lifting and holding *their bosoms. One is sniffing her armpits, wondering if her antiperspirant has POOFED away too.*

Someone shouts: "Oh no, everything's gone! This is not funny!"

Barb rushes to the mirror – "Mirror, mirror on the wall, who the f**k are you?" Without her contact lenses, she is appalled to find that this already blurry apparition staring back at her bears no resemblance to her regal self.

In her cabin, Bee exclaims, "Bloody hell, I've gone from looking older to now looking dug up."

Another shouts, "Has everyone lost all their makeup too, including any trace on their face?"

All respond sarcastically: "Yup, happy days!"

GONG: "Rest assured, queens; we've left you the bare necessities. After all, no woman should be deprived of sanitary wear and hygiene products."

"Phew, there's body butter in this pack. No ashy, itchy skin for me," T is relieved to discover."

Ping notes, "Shower gel and deodorant, but damn it, perfume free."

GONG: "Queens, you will need to form two teams. A tuck box is available for the group. This box contains your rations for the week ahead. It will be replenished next week. Instructions will follow once team selection has taken place."

Ella suggests, "We don't know each other, so the fairest way is to do names out of a hat."

Barb raises what she still thinks is an arched brow and says huffily: "Like that'll work. I propose that I lead one team. Kink, you were the first to step up; you lead the other team."

Kink, having stretched the neckline of her tee shirt, has discovered that by wearing it hanging off one bare shoulder, she can best show off her graceful neck and collarbones. "That's fine, but I'll choose my team first. Ping, I like the look of your pixie cut; you're with me. T, I love the braids; you're in my team."

Barb turns to her team. "Bee, Ella, looks like you're in the winning squad."

GONG: "Queens, Time to face the first challenge – **Seek to take control**. Here are your instructions. You'll receive a map of the island and a list of ingredients to forage. These will be used to make a magic potion. This potion will adapt for the user to either boost (for vitality), ease (provide relief) and/or heal (for strength and restoration). The first team to find all the ingredients may enjoy the potion's benefits."

Tapping her fingers together and squinting to see her team better, Barb says, "We've got this; potions are my thing. Alchemy rules."

Bee worriedly remarks, "Let's not get ahead of ourselves. There had better not be any sodding hills on this island. Not a big climber."

Ella comforts, "Don't worry, we'll look after each other."

Barb has just spotted Kink's perky and bouncy boobs in her now adjusted attire and quickly knots her t-shirt under her tiny but still firm breasts. All the better to show off her slim waistline and still-toned abs. "Trust me; I know what's best for this group. No one chokes on my watch."

Meanwhile, preoccupied with the equipment and the tuck box, Kink's team has apportioned the rations for the week.

Bee is dismayed to see that there's no alcohol in their rations. "Not even a bottle of Prosecco. How will I get through this beastly day, let alone three weeks with this lot."

After a few days of settling in and pleasantries over, they make satisfactory progress in their quest to source potion ingredients. The queens have tackled all obstacles with gusto, but now team Barb finds themselves at the edge of a cliff. They must abseil down to retrieve a magic egg nestled in a crevice below. Queen Bee is terrified. Her team is on hand with ropes and encouragement to ensure her safety. Slowly; they lower her down. With Barb giving clear directions and Ella as the anchor, Bee is stable and successfully retrieves the egg.

Team Kink has taken a different route. Their magic egg sits lower, so they climb up from the base of the cliff. A divide-and-conquer approach is needed. Ping, looking very athletic, climbs up as far as she can go and shouts up to Kink, who waits at the top: "Kink, Kink, let down your binding rope," before grabbing on and climbing up the rest of the way. Their egg is safely retrieved and passed to T, who is in charge of their stash.

Fast forward to the end of the week, and team Barb has successfully collected all of the ingredients for the magic potion. Kink's team is one ingredient short. This sweet victory belongs to team Barb. Then, with a POOF, the ingredients disappear, and a magic potion materialises.

GONG: "The victorious must distribute the potion as they see fit. A little goes a long way."

Queen Barb decides for her team. "Our needs are greater; let's keep the advantage." The tone is set; trouble brews.

In their cabins, two of the queens have noticed that their once shiny copper-framed mirror is slowly gaining patches of green and blue, and their reflection is clearing.

Kink finds herself in front of the mirror and is shocked when it says to her: "I see you, be careful."

"Appreciate the sentiment, but A TALKING MIRROR! C'mon."

Over at Ping's cabin, she's also noting similar discolouration's to her mirror. It, too, is clearing. It speaks, "For too long, you've trusted only yourself; there's value in team play."

"But we lost. Not sure I'm brave enough to trust others," says Ping.

Start of week two.

*GONG: "The wheel of chance with a menu of modern-day tweakments awaits in the communal area. Each queen will have a turn to spin for the promise of an enhancement. Warning: this is a game of **Good intentions with uncertain outcomes**. The spell lasts for the duration of this camp. So what have you got to lose? How lucky are you feeling?"*

Bee – "This is not my first rodeo, ladies. Look and learn. She steps up, spins the wheel, and ... POOF!"

No one notices any changes at first, but then she smiles and is practically luminous. Her already whitened teeth have had a double dose of whitening, and her now oversized veneers have distorted her smile. Someone sniggers, another whispers, "Goofy lives."

Next up is Ping, who ideally would prefer laser hair removal. She spins the wheel, and POOF finds herself with long and luscious hair extensions. "Ridiculous," she tuts as she marches away.

Kink spins the wheel with an eye on the teeth combo treatment: correction and whitening. POOF, her forehead starts to prickle, and her eyebrows shoot up and remain in place. She's finding it hard to blink. She turns to the group. "Botox?"

"Why look so surprised?" says Barb, sniggering.

Tension mounts within the group. It's anyone's guess what the naughty wheel will deliver next. "It's making a mockery of us."

Resignedly, Ella steps up to the wheel; she sees the hair treatment plan and secretly wishes that the dial will stop there. POOF, Groucho Marx, and micro-bladed brows it is. The group gasps at the result, and Kink exclaims: "Good Lord!"

Barb's up next and hopes that discrete lip fillers will come her way. POOF. Her face tightens, and she clutches her already chiselled jaw. Her now thread-lifted jawline and the group's collective gasp tells her that she resembles Munch's painting 'The Scream.'

Bella, by this stage, knows what's coming. POOF, and sure enough, her already plump lips start inflating slowly. She can already feel her inner lip drying. "Well, thish ish a bit of a shitsh show," she lisps.

Three days pass, and both teams feel hard done by. They are still adjusting to their misfired tweakments. Back in the communal hut, Bee is hangry. Her portion size has been severely restricted, and her pick-me-up comfort foods are not part of their daily rations. She doesn't realise that her clucking's and banging's are attracting the attention of others.

"Why so glum Glow-in-the-dark? What are you cussing about?" Asks Ping.

"All right for you to say Pongy, but I'm STARVING!" Bee spits.

"Now, let's play nice. Kindness wins the day," Ella chimes in.

"Shut it, Grouch-Ella. This is not the time to tra-la-la." Barb retorts.

And yet Team Barb, with their daily dose of the magic potion, still shows a can-do approach to any tasks. Initial gallows humour subsides into a drumbeat of resentment amongst Team Kink. Without the magic potion's benefits, they feel distinctly disadvantaged as they go about their daily tasks.

Kink has been snorkelling. The others watch her emerging from the surf. Her white tee shirt clinging to her buoyant breasts, the side-to-side locomotion of her hips entrancing her audience. Seduction complete, she thinks smugly and slides her mask over her head—the group titters.

"What's the joke?" Kink asks.

"You are," they chime. T explains, "You look like you've sheen shome-thing shcary, amushing, or both. Hard to tell."

GONG. "Queens, the rest of this week is all about arduous work. An-other challenge - **Drudge without glory.** The task is to fill two large vats with pure water from the waterfall located on the other side of the island. By the end of the week, the vat with the purest drinking water has con-quered the quest, and the reward is an early reversal of the tweakments."

As Kink watches Team Barb talking excitedly amongst themselves, practically skipping to collect their buckets, she says menacingly, "This will be hard for us. I think it's time to get dirty."

"Ish that a shuggeshtion, or a proposhal? We can't tell anymore," lisps T nervously.

"It's no laughing matter; I'm serious. I mean it." Growls Kink.

T and Ping disagree with her. "No. Trust us, dirty tricks don't work. Hard effort pays off. It's all we've ever known."

But Kink still wants that victory. It's payback time for not sharing the potion.

The game commences, and armed with their buckets, they all start the trek. Back and forth, back and forth, back and forth they go.

"This is beyond dull," says Barb, once again overtaking Team Kink.

"Eashyy for you to shay," lisps T, whilst packing on her ever-diminishing lip balm.

"Let's tap into our inner queens," says Ella, singing, "Something inside so strong, I know that we can take it..."

"Not quite Groucho, tough, not fluff nails it," says Ping, irritated, as she flings her new extensions away from her face.

Ella is blissfully unaware of the middle finger flips of the other team as they pass her.

"Ish she for real?" mutters T grumpily.

Back and forth they go. The harder Team Kink work, the lower their morale. "There may be no "I" in team, but there is certainly an "I" in win," plots Kink as she keeps her head down.

Despite the objections of her teammates, she takes matters into her own hands, and on the night before the finish, under cover of darkness, she muddies the water of the opposing team's vat.

It's the end of the week, and all the queens are exhausted. Even Bee's lip curtain has come down over her luminous gnashers. As dawn breaks, they see yardsticks placed inside each vat, and a ducking stool sits above. Team Kink seeing the levels, realises with dismay that despite their arduous work, they have fallen short. Meanwhile, team Barb is giddy with celebration.

"Are you thinking what I'm thinking?" Ella says to Ping. "Yup, someone is going to get wet,"

GONG: "Queens, gather around the vats. Remember, the challenge was to collect the highest volume of pure drinking water. But not so fast with your celebration; surface level is one thing; now comes the test for clarity.

Time to shake things up. As you chose to remain in teams, it's time to swap your leaders. So, leaders, get on to the opposing team's ducking stool. Your new teammates will administer any punishment."

As she climbs onto her stool, Kink is faced with a dilemma. Does she stay quiet and hope that Barb is plunged, or does she come clean to her new team? On water clarity, she knows that now they don't stand a chance; eventually, dirt ALWAYS gets revealed.

Barb knows that with this switch to the new team, her previous selfish behaviour has put her in jeopardy of a dunking.

The silence of the leaders is deafening. Their guilt is palpable. Their eyes lock, and there's a moment where they recognise that they both have the killer instinct and will stop at nothing to win. But, equally, they think, No one controls me. So simultaneously, they reach for their levers. Then, cackling loudly, they plunge themselves.

After the group's collective gasp, Ella and Bee exclaim, "But why?!" Then as Kink clambers out with her now less-than-white attire, it becomes clear to all what's transpired.

"Oh no, she did it after all," Ping says in dismay.

"We're shtuck with theesh tweakmentsh." says T sadly.

"Why did it have to be two teams?" says Bee.

"I don't think it said that. We all just assumed," says Ping.

"Sho, we could have worked together, rather than againsht each other," exclaims T, as the penny drops. With that recognition, POOF: All the tweakments immediately reverse.

Surprised and with sighs of relief, they return to their cabins. They are delighted to find their vanity cases back in place.

In T's cabin, her mirror speaks: "You can see what others fail to see. Now recognise the value in yourself." Her mirror's frame gains the same beautiful patina.

Start of week three.

GONG: "Queens, good morning. Another week ahead. Please assemble in the meeting hut."

The tinkling sound of chitter chatter precedes their arrival as a now familiar group. It's immediately obvious that they feel more at ease with themselves and each other. It's also apparent that the potion has been shared across the group. Those who wear make-up have dialled down considerably, wearing the bare minimum for comfort. All have nourished skin, and some are wafting pleasant scents. Two weeks of eating healthily and moving with purpose are beginning to show. They feel less creaky and cranky. They're all sleeping well, and without the stresses of their public life, they are now wearing a face of contentment and vitality.

GONG: "Queens, this week may be your most challenging week yet. The challenge is **RAW to ROAR**. It will assess your physical, mental, and emotional boundaries. However, the rewards are worth playing for. Three obstacles await: One to pass through, one to pass under, and one to pass over. Every obstacle will need collaboration. This challenge takes place midweek. Until then, use your time wisely."

"What can it be?" they are thinking.

"I'm up for anything, as long as it's fun," says Bee excitedly.

"As long as I'm not caged," fears Kink.

"No group hugs for me," says Barb dismissively.

"Being muted, as usual," thinks Tee.

"Whatever it is, it must have clear rules," says Ping.

"And nobody gets hurt," says Ella.

With three days to go, they're left to ponder the next challenge.

"What do we do in the meantime?" asks Ping.

"Let's just do our own thing," says Kink as she picks up her mask and snorkel. "Coming, Ping?"

The next day, as the sun sets, Ella grabs her yoga mat and wanders off to find a quiet space. She's surprised to see Barb setting up her mat under the next palm tree. "Ashtanga?" she asks.

"No, Vinyasa," replies Barb as she slides gracefully into a downward-facing dog. Trouble starts when she's doing floorwork, and she moves from 'happy baby' to 'plough' and lets rip.

"Goes with the territory," laughs Ella, and sure enough, with her next move, she trumpets too. "Oops, sorry."

Barb laughs, "And that was sustained."

By now, they're both rolling with laughter.

"Imagine ten years down the line," says Ella.

"If I am still this flexible in ten years, to hell with the explosions. I'll make it more musical." Says Barb.

The following day Bee is up early and sees T wandering around camp.

"You hungry?"

"STARVING!"

"Shall we forage?"

They stumble across a mango tree laden with fruit. With the promise of taking some back for the group, they feel obliged to taste a few too many. With their sweet tooth satiated and sticky with sweet nectar, they lay on the ground clutching full stomachs. Unfortunately, this disturbs a nest of fire ants underneath. Yelping in pain, they hastily fling off their clothes as they dash into the sea. The two snorkellers gain an eyeful of things they now can never unsee.

The conversation around the firepit that evening leads to mirth and more disclosures.

"Kink, tell us, did you see anything interesting snorkelling today?"

"A couple of grey-bearded mussels, a few low-lying clams, and a not-so-cheeky anemone, or four," she replies, nodding slowly.

"Really?" asks Ping. But a wink from Kink answers her query. Suddenly they all get it, and belly laughs follow.

"Let's be honest, over time, change happens in those areas too," laughs Ella.

They all agree. With just one question like "Do you find ...?" suddenly, more embarrassing tales of the change are disclosed.

The group continues to bond.

Later that evening, back in her cabin, Ella's mirror changes and speaks. "Make a friend of time. Wear your age with pride."

Midweek

GONG: "At the start of the boot camp, level one stripped you of all your vanity products, forcing you to go barefaced. You are more than halfway through this camp, and a new level of exposure awaits—time to dig deep."

POOF, three obstacle courses appear behind the communal hut.

The queens survey the terrain ahead and, in unison, huff loudly, "You have got to be kidding!"

*GONG: "Queens. These three obstacles represent the components of your celebrations at the end of this week. All obstacles will need to be completed as a team. Obstacle one is labelled '**No Harm Done**' and exposes your team's constraints and diverse approaches. Good luck."*

Ping steps up and says, "Right, let's do a recce and work out what this is all about. We will need to go low, head down, and squeeze under those barbed wires," she says.

"But it's so muddy and a long way to wriggle through."

"Kiss goodbye to your clean whites."

"Let's just get it over and done with."

They go down. Some queens prefer to wriggle through on their stomachs, thus protecting their ample bosoms and hair. Bottoms get snagged, hair gets pulled, chins scraped, and necks ache. Disliking the taste of mud as they travail.

"Ouch, ouch, the puppies are struggling."

Others have committed to going on their back, and it's tougher. Without any direction, some collide, feet lose purchase and fling mud in the face of those coming up behind, elbows are sore, and shoulders start aching.

"F**k, this is cruel. 'No harm done.' My arse is saying something different."

One by one, they emerge covered in mud, almost unrecognisable. With the initiation obstacle completed, they feel ready to take on the next one.

GONG: "Queens. Well done. Obstacle two is labelled **'Push Through, No U Turns'** *and will have you face your fear and trust in the process to pull through. Once again, good luck."*

"What have we got here?" asks Ping peering over the edge of a vast muddy pond. "And what's the screen across the middle?"

"So no one can see what's on the other side?"

"It looks deep and so very muddy."

"Looks bloody cold!"

"Ok, I'll go first, to see or rather feel what it's all about." She jumps in and disappears for far too long. The tension mounts. Finally, she emerges. They can hear her, but they can't see her. Ripples of relief run across the group. She clambers out on the other side and starts vocally relaying back over the screen. "It's tough but ..."

She's interrupted.

"What's the rope for?" shouts Barb.

"Oh shit, there's a rope?" shouts back Ping. "Damn, I can't swim back; it's a one-way channel. I guess that rope needed to come through with me then. I just didn't see it."

Panic erupts. They realise the rope is their safety and guide.

"Ok, let's think."

"I'm a good swimmer, I'll take it," says Kink, grabbing one end and jumping in. "You hold onto the other end, Barb." She swims through, joining Ping on the other side.

Kink shouts, "I'm through! We'll hold steady here, Barb. You're the anchor there, ok?"

"Yep, ok," Barb shouts back.

"It should be easy now," Ping instructs. "Just use the rope to guide you through. Keep going forward. We must do this one at a time as long as we feed back to help each other. Who's next?"

"I'm not going to overthink. I may lose my nerve. You can do this, Bee," mutters Bee to herself. Then, with a loud gasp, she enters the water and minutes later, she safely emerges on the other side. "I'm through," she shouts back to the others.

Having seen it's possible, T follows suit, and after a while, she yells back. "Safe!"

Ella, whose next in line, looks at Barb and notices, "You're terrified, aren't you?"

Barb admits, "It hurts feeling vulnerable. Honestly, this is a leap of faith for me. I feel like I'm going into the unknown here. I've only ever trusted myself. I need a minute. You go ahead."

Ella hesitates. She's reluctant to leave Barb behind. "I can bring up the rear. Would you like to swap?"

Barb insists, "No, please, you go ahead. In this instance, I'm counting on you to pull me through."

Ella goes through and finally shouts, "I'm through. Barb. Signal when you're ready."

To herself, she chants, "C'mon, Barb, don't panic; you can trust them." But she doesn't trust herself, so as an extra measure, she ties the rope around her waist.

"We've got you, Barb," shouts Kink from the other side.

"F**k it!" she thinks as she tugs the rope and jumps into the water.

Splash.

With everyone safely across, the teams are hoarse with their whoops of joy. And contrary to previous protestations, they do enjoy a group hug.

Soggy but elated the group makes their way to the third and final obstacle: It's a colossal, sloped climbing wall.

"Holy shit, that's monumental!"

GONG: "Queens. Once again, very well done. Another component in the bag. Your final obstacle is labelled **'Getting Over the "Now What?" Hump Together.'** This is all about playing to your strengths, conquering the ascent, and, more importantly, planning your descent. Good luck and see you on the other side."

"How will we ever get to the top?"

"There'll be a way. Can you see the footholds?"

"But look how far apart they are. I'm not stretchy. And I have no upper body strength; how will I hold on?"

"Never mind the ascent; what the hell is waiting for us on the other side?"

"One thing at a time. Let's do this bit first and then reassess," says Ping.

"This is going to need a human pyramid. Who will be the base, and who climbs?" asks Kink.

Without much discussion, they naturally find their places in the pyramid. It was easier than they thought. Ping starts the ascent.

"Didn't think it was going to be this up close and personal."

"Grab on."

"Give me your hand. Hold on."

"Your foot on my shoulder, and I'll shove your bum."

"Oof, nearly there."

Ping summits and straddles the hump. Ella soon joins her. Their quiet assessment of the sheer drop speaks volumes.

"Uh oh."

Kink scrambles up, peers over, and spots three dangling ropes. Undaunted, she knows exactly what needs to be done. "I'm an old hand at this. We can rappel down or knot the ropes for a slower descent. Either way, we won't freefall. I'll show you how to knot." Ping agrees but suggests, "Let's leave one rope unknotted. One for a speedy descent, two for a measured descent."

Using the unknotted rope, Kink swiftly brings it through her legs, across her body, over her right shoulder, and under her armpit into her left hand. Then, pulling it tight, she confidently steps forward while controlling the speed of her descent.

"I'll be down to stabilise the ropes. I can instruct from there."

The pair on the hump exclaim, "Wow! That's impressive; you know what you're doing."

T and Barb are next to be pulled up to the hump. Using Kink's method, Gutsy Ping has already started her descent. Rapidly she joins Kink. Barb reaches down and pulls Bee up into position.

With Kink and Ping securing the ropes, Barb and T choose the knotted descent. Slowly and steadily, hand over hand, leaning out, they walk down the wall.

"Hallelujah, we're safe," says T, who had been holding her breath the entire time.

With neither feeling maverick, Bee and Ella agree to go down the slower-knotted ropes together.

They touch down to a round of applause. It was all about overcoming individual limitations.

GONG: "Queens. That was impressive. Congratulations. Quest complete; the final component is in the bag—a time for celebration. Freshen up; it's time to feast."

Later, Barb comes out of the shower and unconsciously wipes the steamed mirror. She's shocked to discover that her mirror has cleared, but the frame is tarnished. "Damn!"

The mirror speaks: "You look different, softer, kinder. Kindness suits you. Was it so hard to show vulnerability?"

Meanwhile, Bee's mirror speaks to her too. "Don't write yourself off yet; you contribute. There's plenty of life in the old girl yet."

Shocked, "Who said that?" she asks, and the now blue-green framed mirror replies softly, "You did."

At the final campfire, they're all feeling satiated and very sanguine. Ping asks, "Has anyone else's mirror turned from shiny copper to streaks of blue and green?"

All replied. "Yes!"

"I thought with the lights out, it was going mouldy," says Barb.

T says, "The glass has cleared, but the frame is getting more colour."

"Like age spots?" teases Kink.

"No, it's becoming more ...fascinating," sighs Ella.

The next day and the end of the Fiery Queen boot camp.

GONG: "Queens, go well, but finally, please remember to retrieve your mirror from your cabin and take it home with you. It keeps you safe. After all, a speaking mirror is useless to anyone else but you."

Mirrors are safely retrieved, and the Queens are gathered in the communal hut before departure. They are surprised that no one mirror is the same. Every mirror is different in size and shape.

All the mirrors are exquisite in daylight, a Verdigris patina with distinctly different blue, green, and copper streaks, heralding a new beginning.

GONG: "Queens, henceforth, celebrate the present you and let go of the past."

The only thing the mirrors had in common was an inscription at the bottom.

'You are good enough!'

THE END

And that, dear listeners, concludes the tale of the feary to fiery warrior queens, from RAW to ROAR.

Ultimately, these queens were more accepting of themselves and each other—a lesson to us all. Let's hope they keep their sisterhood strong. There are still many battles lying ahead in their realms.

The Queens' new charter for the individual is to remember:

1. Beauty starts with health.
2. Beauty is tarnished by bad behaviour.
3. Function matters more than form.
4. Support each other, do not compete.
5. No bias

The Queens' new charter for the beauty industry is transparency:

1. Safety (no harmful ingredients)
2. Ethical
3. No animal cruelty
4. Sustainable
5. Culturally appropriate
6. Affordable essential hygiene
7. No false claims & misleading advertising

GONG: "Thank you, Queens. Job done."

| 13 |

India's story

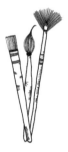

'Free range dogs and low flying children' is the sign in the drive of our house.

I have overheard the cleaners and gardeners describe our home as "Posh Feral." Hugo and I smile. This setting is exactly what we have strived to achieve; a stylish home yet relaxed.

The building itself is beautiful with idyllic grounds. Internally we have refurbished it with up-to-the-minute technology, and modern Italian furnishings, all peppered with treasured antiques. Overall, visitors have said it has an air of old money, an understated elegance. The most important thing for us is that it is primarily a home; and not a showpiece. Having said that, it can polish up quite nicely if so required.

Life in our home is chaotic, with trip-worthy toys and comfort blankets strewn across many floors. All of this indicates that our breeding endeavours have been successful. However, Hugo and I were lonely as children and overlooked by more favoured siblings. Our parents were too interested in their careers and escapades. I certainly felt more of a second thought than the golden child.

Thus, when Hugo and I got together, we agreed to have a large family, to create a dynasty of our own. And so we did.

Six children came along easily, one after the other, all healthy, cherished bundles of joy. Fascinatingly, each child was quite different from the other: different coloured eyes; different coloured hair; different levels of cheekiness; but *all* with lovely easy-going characters. The gene pool was the same: same parents, so the same mixture but unique buns came out of the oven. I marvelled at every one of them. As I predicted, at least one was a redhead. Phoebe's blonde hair turned increasingly red. She would become a titian blonde, a renaissance girl, like me. Later, our redhead boy, Felix, was in a different league on the red scale. He was a dark 'copper top.' A Duracell battery with dynamo energy to match. If his hair grew too long at school, they would mock him as 'Ronnie McDonald.' But, contrary to the clichéd views of redheads being hot-tempered, Felix was the opposite, always slow to react. He just shrugged off any intended hurt and continued to blaze a trail of fun and joy, with perhaps the occasional calamity

Felix was a charmer, mischievous and bright. He got himself out of trouble most of the time. Only once did he need my help. If boisterous play caused damage to other people's property, Hugo and I would throw money at the incident. Compensate for peoples' losses and simply buy the family out of trouble. Felix knew without a shadow of a doubt that we had his back, no matter what. He wore this confidence effortlessly. I celebrated him daily. The magic of the Felix effect was indefinable. It made him instantly popular and memorable. I so wish I had had that as a child. Instead, back then, I found comfort in drawing and losing myself in my imaginary worlds.

Having been overlooked in my own family, I don't believe in favourites, and despite the comet of the red boy, our children all know that. We see them, we value them, and we celebrate their differences. It's a perpetual if not relentless, task. Yet they all have their view of my preferences. Sibling rivalry needs to be kept in check constantly. I am also aware that, of course, I identify with the titian blonde, eye-catching hair of Phoebe and the outrageously red hair of Felix. I love all of them equally; I identify with the outstanding and limiting aspects of being a red. They both have my skin: too -pale, almost translucent and with a fine dappling of freckles. I made it clear from the outset that they needed to protect their skin from the sun, as they would burn. But, of course, they had to experience the pain and discomfort more than once to realise the value of my warning

I often reflect that if I had been mousy, I might have had quite a different path; unremarkable and bland. Instead, my glorious mane of strawberry blonde hair sets me apart and has attracted many admirers. People are fascinated with it because it is glossy rather than frizzy. My Mother expressed relief - as if she would have sent me back if my colouring had been paler. "At least you're not insipid, darling," she would say, which sounded like that would have been a crime.

Despite my toad of a brother, I find boys straightforward. As a child, when invited, I could always rough and tumble with the best of them. My ball skills garnered respect from the village boys. Amusingly, without me, they would get told off for breaking the rules. I loved climbing trees, scrambling over fences and shooting cans off a wall. But if our gang broke a greenhouse window, I was always let off for being a girl. Once this band of mischief-makers recognised this and my ability to sweet talk, they included me more often. This inclusion soon evaporated once hormones raised their ungainly head.

As my body changed in my teens, so too did the boys' gaze. Increasingly I became aware of the power of my sex. When dancing, the boys became incoherent if I accidentally flashed a leg or when a strawberry nipple unintentionally fell out of my dress. It was all a bit of a surprise, a giggle even. That is, with boys my age. It became increasingly alarming when older males came along.

Whilst remaining slender, I grew taller and curvier. At 16, I began attracting attention that I didn't necessarily want. My local boys were still lovely, but some of their new friends were less so. Simon was my first love, and we took things slowly, but when it came to my first act of passion, Simon made it clear that I was a trophy. He said callously, "You're my first redhead." I thought that I had meant something more to him. He had played me. I was hurt and so became overly cautious with the next boyfriend. As lovely as the boys were, yet again, they fixated on my hair. A pattern was evolving with them singling me out to conquer and notch up potentially. My interest in boys was dwindling, and I became uncharacteristically withdrawn until someone recommended dressage. The intimate connection with a powerful animal is where I found my confidence. Horses became my new passion, and I excelled at it. Later if it involved equine sport, I was there—hacking, jumping, and eventually, being part of the local polo team.

I was beginning to think that all my energy, time and money was only ever to be invested in four-legged trusted companions when a proud steed came into view. At a polo match, after a disappointing loss and a clumsy dismount on my part, Hugo came along, offering a glass of champagne. At first, I was on guard; No one would ever chalk me up again. But there was no need to worry. Hugo was a softy, and it turned out he had fallen early and hard. He proved his solid character when on our first date, I drank too much, slipped and did the loudest fart before throwing up over his new shoes. He laughed and said, "Impressive, both ends at once!" I was mortified and wanted the ground to swallow me, but he cleaned me up and quietly dropped me back home. He rang the next day to see if I was all right and to book another date.

The second date was a surprise—a good one, an excellent one. I was sober and remembered everything. We talked. The more Hugo listened, the more I spoke. So back and forth it went, and by the end of the evening, I felt that I'd always known him and that this one deeply understood me. Hugo confessed that, of course, my red hair and the paleness of my skin attracted him initially, but my calm, unflappable character, elegance and modesty cemented his attraction. He fast became my champion when he recognised my brother, with his academic and sporting brilliance, eclipsed me time after time. This same brother who my parents had celebrated, whilst I, with my B grades, which were 'good enough' but not outstanding, had been expected to fall in. So I did. Over the years, my arrogant brother had got away with murder, always favoured and dobbing me in at every opportunity. My parents were oblivious to his spite; to this day, he remains the golden child who could do no wrong. But Hugo noticed because he had been overlooked in his family, like me.

"Where are your wins, your rosettes and trophies? He asked. They were displayed but behind my brother's Polo trophies and rowing cups. "Look closer, behind the frames of the first team players," I replied.

He also registered my skill as an artist but queried why my parents never mentioned my annual wins in art competitions, nor were there any paintings on display in the family home. He pledged to remedy this, and since then, he has done that.

Later, Hugo and I quickly realised that with our children, it was less of what you say and more of what you do when acknowledging their achievements. We have had to work at it. At separate times, an individual would shine. Our efforts have worked by and large; our family is generally secure and happy. On many occasions, they behave as one, supporting and defending each other without question (to anyone outside the family). Naturally, it is a different matter if there is a spat within the ranks.

Hugo has always made me feel special. To him, I was his moon goddess. We are a partnership. We simply get on and feel like each other's corresponding jigsaw piece. As I said, we were, from the start, with one accord, building our little dynasty.

Our wedding was spectacular, with morning suits, top hats for the chaps, and an ethereal copper theme for the flowers, the cake, and my bridesmaids. I wore a champagne-coloured dress with butter-coloured pearls and tried to evoke a Titania in Autumn theme. It caused quite a stir in the village. The country church was decked out in yellow, gold and orange foliage, and a reception followed the sweet service in a marquee. All very expected. The major surprise was a Man of honour rather than a Maid of honour (a male cousin I adored). He was outrageously camp, delighting me in particular, as his campy charm gently ruffled the feathers of my parents. Hugo's parents were surprisingly non-plussed. Another cousin, this time one of Hugo's, turned up with blonde dreadlocks and a straw hat (both of which broke the formal dress code) and raised eyebrows. It was just what we wanted. We had gently stamped our intention of doing things a little differently. My domineering mother wanted to put her mark on everything but was politely ignored by all. We let her keep to her blue, mother-of-the-bride theme, even though it remained in contrast to the rest of the wedding party. Throughout the ceremony, she sulked outrageously before getting ridiculously drunk and being escorted back home by my long-suffering, embarrassed father.

By the time we returned from our honeymoon in the Bahamas, I was pregnant with Phoebe and never to return to work after that. Nevertheless, life in our London home was satisfactory, and the daily coffee gatherings were a gentle start to a lifetime of motherhood. With only one child, I joined every baby event possible: baby massage; baby and mother yoga; chicken pox parties; you name it. It was a succession of rainbow nappy discussions, but maybe the baby cashmere parties were a step too far. It turns out that mashed banana stains cashmere in the same way that it stains something from a recycled charity shop! Hugo questioned some of the yummy mummies' perspectives, and as we wanted a clan, our babies had to forego designer baby wear.

I loved being pregnant. I blossomed and felt invincible. My figure snapped back quickly after the birth, and baby Alastair came along soon after Phoebe. He was my best 30th birthday present. With two young children, I felt wedded to the nursing chair and that these bovine years would forever define me and my breasts! The other city mothers were highly ambitious and, with domestic help, upwardly mobile. I felt the odd one out, I had never been a city girl, and my heart belonged to country life. Being constrained in this bustling city with two young children was more difficult than I thought. This isolation was the worst form of loneliness ever.

Hugo prospered in his early thirties, and his career went from strength to strength in the city. He enjoyed his male mates and gentleman's clubs, sometimes staying out too long and a little too often. He was avoiding those sleepless nights with screaming babies. Even with his constant reassurance and declarations of love, I checked his pockets and sniffed the collars of his work shirts. As the tension in our relationship escalated, I found a hotel receipt for two, which wasn't ours. The row that followed was like none we've had before or since. It turns out that it was his colleague Antony. Liverpool client meeting, overrun, late check-in, only a double available, needs must. Hugo uncharacteristically exploded: "What more do I have to do to convince you? I love YOU. Full stop!"

Later, I overheard him retelling a city friend, "I've got far too much to lose if I even think of fucking it all up, so I won't." I knew then that he would remain faithful.

We enjoy our wealth and feel lucky to have found each other. Not just because we have married well, it was expected. We liked each other too. We took life in our stride, and at the turn of the century, with all its amazing parties, the millennium heralded a bright future for our family. Or so we thought.

The 9/11 event in 2001 propelled Hugo and me to search for a house outside London before Phoebe started school. Cedar House practically winked at us when we had a drive-by. Nestled in its land, it was perfect. The children squealed in chorus to Hugo's excitement. They shared a vision of building a tree house. Something that Hugo had always dreamed of but had been denied. At last, we were moving back to Hampshire. Hugo's sister, Miranda, was also happy we were moving closer to his family.

Miranda could be a bit difficult until you get to know her. But, over the years, we have become good friends and sisters-in-law. The turning point in our relationship was recognising that, as horsewomen, we were evenly matched, despite being hugely different characters.

My love of horses continued to run deep. I've always instinctively connected and communicated with them. Subtle body positioning and strength in my thighs made me a natural rider. It also won quiet admiration, if not surprise, from Miranda. She had clearly written me off in the early days, bar the hair. She thought I was yet another one of Hugo's instantly forgettable fillies. That is until she went out riding with me.

I chose Nero, a stallion known to be a little tricky. I mounted him with ease and grace and set off with absolute confidence. When the horse tried it on, I responded vocally with calm and low commands and squeezed my thighs. He quickly responded and knew he would not get the better of me. I was not to be trifled with. Nero became my favourite horse. We had a special bond. Other riders acknowledged and admired our connection, not least Hugo, who always selected his favourite gentle mare.

Miranda remarked, "You mastered him quickly. Nero, I mean…," to which I replied. "I come in peace. If it's a war between him and me, the loser will not be me. They read our minds don't they?"

Miranda said, "Apparently so,"

I was twenty-five then and thirty-four with the move to Cedar House. With Baby Felix on the way, my re-acquaintance with Nero had to wait. And no sooner had I finished breastfeeding than I became pregnant again. Serious little Rory was on his way. My joints felt like overstretched rubber bands, and I feared I would never get back on a horse. But, silly me, everything eventually returns to how it was. Lesson learned.

Our thirties and forties were busy. Building our home, raising the children, and having a succession of various home helps who came and went. Hugo continued to commute to London, and our country life was filled with children's parties, game shoots, village fetes and the odd corporate party back in the city too, which I managed reasonably well. There were two memorable moments. One - when my boobs leaked through my burnt orange silk dress and the ever-increasing circle that drew the bosses' attention. The second time when a breast pad went AWOL, I had one leaky boob, but it was also lopsided. Sometimes the dinner and speeches were too long, making it difficult to express the surplus milk before seamlessly returning to the table.

When Phoebe turned eleven, it was a milestone for all, but I remember it most for Hugo sulking at turning forty. "The city is a young man's game," he would start saying. I didn't hear the rest of that. I know that my spotlight was fully beamed and focused on our children. Feeling unseen for a while, Hugo started to turn his attention to classic cars, eventually joining an old-timer's club. His joy in restoring old bangers was unbridled. "Plenty of life left in this old girl yet," he declared.

I didn't feel old. I was still fertile, bringing new life into the world. My fortieth birthday present was little blonde Alice with curls and baby blue eyes. I was in heaven. Little did we know then that she would grow into a tomboy, casting Rory aside and becoming Felix's favourite pet. Another change in the family dynamic. Once again, a reminder to me that they're individuals. Without Hugo around, Miranda was my constant companion in and out of the stable yard, usually propping up the Aga, often helping herself to anything in the larder. She was a fixture in our home and a force to be reckoned with. She'd grown to love me, occasionally becoming too familiar, overstepping the mark, and I would need to rein her in. I had to remind her that it was not her roost to rule but Hugo's. Apart from sharing a love of horses, we shared a love of the children, but mostly, we shared the love of Hugo. Miranda still can't resist mocking the pair of us with our intention of populating half of Hampshire, but Hugo and I know that it was always our goal. Anyway, the benefits for a single, child-free Miranda were fun, fun, fun, sharing in their adventures, and spoiling them rotten. And as long as Hugo could finance it, we kept making babies.

But sex wasn't all about making babies. We enjoyed it in all its manifestations. It has evolved as the years have passed. Not as giddy as it was at the start, in our twenties. That was fast and ardent. We couldn't get enough of each other then. Over the years, we have experimented with various, sometimes hilarious, themes, positions, and locations. Even when we were tired, and it was a little brief, even routine, sex was always easy. Hugo and I trusted each other, and we bonded intimately. And, if time allowed, we were still, on occasion, capable of achieving the whole mind, body and soul experience.

Of course, it was interrupted by a succession of pregnancies, all too easily conceived. Essentially each one was trouble-free. Hugo tolerated each pregnancy and the impact it had on us. He was absorbing the financial burden each time. We both navigated the waves of exhaustion with its customary rare but loving sex. Breast-feeding, while difficult, provided another layer of intimacy. Hugo still thought me beautiful and enjoyed tasting the breast milk. Weirdly, that was such a turn-on. I never wanted that feeling to stop.

With its perpetual movement from conception to weaning, Motherhood altered my internal status from invisible to invincible. It was helped by the fact that I didn't suffer from morning sickness and that my hair, skin and nails flourished. I felt myself bloom each time. But was this just vanity or a mother earth complex?

Or maybe it's much deeper than that? I never felt alone when carrying another human being inside me. A midwife told me that most women know when they've had their last baby. I wondered when that would be. After each of my natural deliveries, the hormonal rush and the post-climactic euphoria that followed were on par with my most incredible orgasms. Procreation had a chemistry of its own.

Growing our family meant we had to expand our support team. Home help around the house proved to be a Godsend. There was a lengthy period where it felt as though there was one au pair after another, each bringing with them their rituals and traditions and leaving with their emotional baggage. It made for a hectic household. But Lord knows how we could function without this support.

There was never a year without a mild drama of one sort or another: quick flights to A&E; au pairs had their hearts broken by various suitors; unjust scores in winter rugby and summer cricket matches. But the home remained largely safe and happy—no scandal within, just casualties out. Our household was thriving.

After the fifth child, I had an unexpected miscarriage. It was early in the pregnancy. The embryo had passed quickly; before the 12 weeks were up, there was no need to tell anyone. Hugo cradled me in his arms and let me quietly sob. My heart was caving in and physically aching. The only other profound loss I could recall was Bramble, my first pony, a Shetland, put down without my consent. He was old but not ready to go yet. He was my first animal love. Mother had swiftly called the vet to put him down before telling me, before I could assess, and before I could say goodbye.

Similarly, this miscarriage brought that helpless fête accompli feeling back again. Yes, it was a shock. Again, I felt denied, helpless and robbed.

The second miscarriage stunned both of us. It was later than 12 weeks; we had already told a few friends. After the spotting, a scan confirmed that the foetus was not viable. I could either surgically remove the contents of conception or allow my body to pass it naturally. I elected for the latter. Thinking that it was not imminent, I continued life as usual. It was winter, thank goodness, and I had several layers on. The bleed started in a coffee shop— NO warning, followed by the whoosh. I whispered to my friend. "It's happening." She offered to drive me to the hospital, but I knew what to expect and insisted on going home. As I stepped out of her car, to my horror, it was like a scene from that Tarantino film, 'Reservoir of Dogs.' My friend stayed with me throughout, but the bleeding continued too long. Panicking, she rang Hugo. I could hear her describing it as a blood bath. Hugo was instantly alarmed, and he was on his way. By the time he got home, the bleeding had subsided, and that's when he got angry. But as I stood up off the loo, I fainted. He carried me to bed and sat with me. He cried; I couldn't. I was numb and exhausted but felt terror in the pit of my stomach: an ache for the baby that was.

We were both frightened by the experience. That time I was much further along in the pregnancy, and the miscarriage was a much bigger deal. Hugo avoided having sex for a while, as now he viewed it as having scary consequences. The later pregnancies changed his perspective. They were now fraught with more risks than joy. We had been complacent. He discussed the realisation of ageing with me, but I disregarded his words. I became depressed. Our doctor agreed with Hugo's comments about problems with geriatric mothers and the increased risks. That didn't help at all. The doctor was very matter-of-fact, only redeeming himself when he referred me to a counsellor. Hoorah! The counsellor was female and listened. Then she truly listened, enabling me to grieve and finally accept the loss.

There was still that need that felt like unfinished business. I resolved to get strong and healthy to ride again. The fitter I became, the less Hugo or anyone else would write me off as geriatric any-thing. For Hugo, this last miscarriage was a game-changer, but the game plan hadn't changed for me. I would get checked out and convince him to try again. This time, to complete every seat at our table. I would have to be more sensitive to his needs. Play to his desire without the spectre of risk and responsibility. I would bear that.

I'll admit it; I set out to seduce my husband. I started dabbling again. Out came the easel, canvas, and brushes, and this time I featured the hidden curves of the female form. As a car enthusiast, Hugo was bound to have his interest piqued. He was getting excited at the smell of turpentine and oil again. No talk of babies, just rampant sex for the fun of it. And sure enough, there was a new lease of life in our bedroom and bathroom.

Sex throughout any fertile month had a score of its own anyway. Hot and urgent when I was on heat, some days going through the motions and surprisingly aroused, then transactional, faking orgasm to get it done.

However, I still had to navigate the bath time dilemma. I've always wondered what it is about men that when you've taken a relaxing bath, having smelled the exotic aromas, become aroused, immediately want to mess it all up, soil you, and then leave you to sleep in *their wet patch.*

Over the last few years, I have choreographed the bath time / sex time dance to a T. Satisfying all concerned and expertly securing my 'me' time.

It went like this.

I would run the bath deliberately too hot, leave it, take a shower, and orchestrate sex. Then after Hugo's climax, we'd talk about anything important (because that is when he truly listens). Then, I'd return to the aromatherapy bath, knowing he would be contentedly asleep. Finally, I went to bed. Brilliant. Everyone was satisfied.

My 'no mention babies' seduction plan had worked. Hugo was now seeing me again as a woman, not a mother. But while my ardour was getting harder, he was beginning to struggle. He put it down to stress and possibly one snifter too many. I feared that we were starting to be out of sync.

Then on the night of my multimedia art exhibition, in the village hall, bingo! I found out I was pregnant. More importantly, the pregnancy was going to hold. I kept it quiet for as long as possible. Hugo was engaged in a very intense work project; he didn't notice that I hadn't been riding for a while. I wouldn't chance any stumble or poor footing of horse or rider impacting my last shot at motherhood. Finally, when fourteen weeks were up, I requested a private scan, and when all was clear, I revealed the new baby on its way to Hugo. He was delighted if a little weary and said, "Ok, last one."

I was relieved but noted the finality of his statement.

Baby number six was an easy and fast birth. A shock of black ebony hair was the only surprise. She was healthy and loud. We welcomed little Maddie with relief and joy into the world. All indulged her. We had done it. I felt blessed, dare I say, a little smug. We had three healthy boys and three healthy girls. Yet a nagging realisation of time running out remained. It had me wondering: who will I be when my baby-making factory inevitably closes?

When I said, in the moment that I could go again, Hugo's resounding, "Absolutely not, I'm getting the snip!" was like a slap around the face. Decision made. It was final. I should be grateful, but it was still hard-hitting at a time when I felt raw. It silenced me.

Maddie was a dream baby, soon sleeping through the night. So after my eight-week check-up with the doctor, who told me my horse riding could resume within the year. Being back in the saddle was part of the tapestry of my life.

When I think back, the intervening years have had a few notable events that registered the growth of our family. Phoebe was going through a crisis with her GCSEs and her first heartbreak. There was no doubt that the older boys were sexually developing, albeit at different stages. Then, one summer, a new sexy Spanish Au pair came to stay. The musky and pungent smell of their rooms became overwhelming. It was a relief when she left.

One Guy Fawkes night, my father suddenly dropped dead from a heart attack, and from then on, my mother became more needy (but still wouldn't offer to help with childcare). Maybe because of my father's death, I cracked a virgin tooth (unfilled) and had my first and only crown installed.

I am now accustomed to the insult of wearing reading glasses, having taken for granted my 20: 20 vision until then. At forty-five, it was as if someone had flipped a switch. It felt like personal decay was knocking. Suddenly I couldn't read food labels. Putting various food industry conspiracies behind me, I struggled to read the labels and booked an eye test. My vision had changed; all perfectly normal. The optometrist made it clear that these things happen at my age. Thanks! The reassurance didn't stop it from being irksome that I couldn't be without my face furniture. I chose the most stylish, amber-framed pair. Hugo reluctantly admitted that he also needed reading glasses (deemed essential for work), especially when reading the Sunday Papers. Irritatingly, he kept picking up mine, so I populated most rooms with cheap spare pairs.

At around this time, Felix started boarding school, and a bully instantly targeted him. I knew it was inevitable. Rupert, his nemesis, made his presence known from the start. There were many threats, a few too many shoves and 'accidental' knocks, all of which left bruises. However, when questioned about his time at school, he dismissed any enquiry and said he could handle it. Indeed Felix was growing strong, but I worried. The rugby pitch was becoming a constant battlefield, and that was just within its own side. When we attended matches, I found myself counting the marks on his face and body.

One day, we got a call from the school. The headmaster's PA said Felix was to be collected immediately; he had been suspended. When we asked what had happened, she said that our son had knocked a boy unconscious and that the hospital was assessing him for concussion. When we arrived, Felix explained that despite his avoidance, Rupert had continued to verbally goad and physically shove him into walls when no one else was around until one day, Felix snapped. He had had enough. "So I hit him bloody hard, and I'm not sorry!" he protested. He was suspended for two weeks until the end of the term. The headmaster said the usual reprimands but without much conviction.

Sometimes bullies need to be on the receiving end of a punishment to make them think twice in future. Felix said that he wasn't worried; he and Rupert had an understanding now but warned that Rupert's mother was a nightmare, "She won't let this go."

I agreed with my son, I had already registered Rupert's mother, Ruth, as one of the mums to avoid. So I walked away whenever I could. I find the 'Ruth's' of this world a bit sad, really. I was mainly non-communicative whenever we met at the touchline or on any of the other school occasions. In those early days, Ruth would always sidle up, ask too many questions, gossip unkindly and offer snide remarks. I think Ruth found me forgettable, dull probably.

She doesn't think so anymore. At the boys' next match, true to form, her vicious slander began. There was no doubt that it was aimed at Felix. I was ready for her. I had chosen to wear my jodhpurs and had taken my crop, yet I had no intention of riding that day, Hugo queried my attire, and I said, "Because I felt like it." Watching the abuse continue unabatedly, I strode across to Ruth in her clucking group. Stretched to my full height, I asked to have a quiet word and when at almost kissing distance, I calmly and briefly delivered what I had to say. She conceded and retreated to her group. Enough of this nonsense, I thought. Hugo was curious and asked what I had said to her. I replied, "I'll tell you later." I never did. He announced to the kids, "Never underestimate your mother; she's a tigress," for a while, in front of the kids, when heading off to various parents' meetings together, he would say, "Come along, stripy."

The only other recollection of this period was one of Miranda's favourite tales when we took on a bully together. It was just the pair of us riding out when we came across a grey without its rider. We picked up the reins and took her back to the yard. The muddy, clearly thrown rider put down his mug of tea and approached his horse. He thanked us for bringing her back, but when we were out of earshot, or so he thought, he proceeded to take his crop and whip the mare in a fury, shouting obscenities.

Miranda quickly turned, and rode back, indeed rode at him, screaming, "What the hell are you doing? No wonder she threw you; you should be dog meat!" She was incandescent and dangerous. I, too, was outraged but could see the situation becoming very nasty. So I dismounted, got in between them and said to him calmly, "Sir, I have a proposition for you. If this is your horse and you are simply incompatible, I'll buy her from you. I'll leave my name and number at the stables. They know me; think about it."

He was still petulant, if a little wary. Silent for a minute, he said, "Ok, I'll think about it." I mounted my horse again, and Miranda and I rode off. She didn't share my belief in the guy's acquiescence. To her, he was "just an arrogant shit. You're wasting your time." I shared her view, but for the horse's sake, the man needed an exit route to save his pride. Some weeks later, Miranda was surprised when Hugo told her we had acquired a lovely grey called 'Pretty Penny' for one of the children. Like her brother, I am true to my word.

"Ah! So that's where my Penny came from," said Rory.

I remember when Penny joined our paddock because that was the time I noticed that my hair had enough grey coming through to accept that it was time to visit the hairdressers. My mane was my signature. Its colour was one thing, but the gloss in my hairline at the front had diminished, and it was beginning to frizz in damp weather. I became obsessed with hair masks. Towards the end of my forties, in disbelief, I found two grey pubic hairs raising their ugly heads. Immediately, I shaved it all off—time to be pubescent again. Hugo was less keen on my bald approach, claiming he liked a patch to determine which way was up in the dark. I teased that he didn't visit that area often enough to complain.

Hugo, in general, was frequently mentioning various disappointments and irritations. He was now at the top of his career ladder- a success by anyone's standard. It didn't make sense. I hoped he wouldn't become a grumpy older man. I noticed he was easily flattered by young women but never doubted his commitment to me. I just wondered if he still desired me. He was always tired and not really in the mood for sex. On the other hand, I wanted sex more than ever, at the very least, to be cuddled and touched.

When Hugo turned fifty in the summer, I threw him an amazingly, lavish ball. We decorated the large barn in the grounds. The weather was great, and our guests arrived to flowers and torches lighting the driveway and to the tune of bagpipes as they alighted from their cars. There were jugglers, fire-eaters, magicians visiting each table, a live band, fireworks and a kedgeree breakfast before 'carriages at dawn.' I danced all night, and when the last taxi left, much to my dismay, Hugo went straight to bed. I stayed up talking to our house guests. I felt abandoned and more than a little fed up without his presence. Everyone had made so much effort for his benefit, but he kept saying he "felt a bit flat". It didn't help that apparently, I was flirting with everyone. I thought I was a good hostess. So why was he consistently being grumpy and disapproving? After all, there is only one calendar year between us. I had that sense of fear in my stomach again. I needed him.

Around this time, Miranda popped by. Again, it was Hugo that she had called in to speak about. She was worried. On more than one occasion, she had thought he was beginning to doubt himself and feel 'less than.' He'd mentioned that all the young bucks at work, whilst admiring, were increasingly challenging him.

I agreed with her. Hugo did look permanently stressed and tired.

I said that I'd been concerned, too, but felt helpless. Hugo never wanted to talk in-depth about work or anything that troubled him personally, including what was becoming increasingly clear: his erectile dysfunction.

Maybe that's why lately, our sex life was infrequent, brief and goddamn, left me wanting.

It reminded me of a scene from a charming sitcom in my youth, 'Just Good Friends,' when the ageing parents of one of the protagonists have a Sunday afternoon romp. The hen-pecked father turns to his disdainful wife and tentatively seeks reassurance, "Same old magic, Darling?' to which his wife rolls her eyes and replies with a drawn-out sigh, "Same old wand!"

It was funny on television but not so funny now.

If stress was killing our sex life, perhaps it was time to get away for a romantic weekend of re-kindling. The challenge was to find the gap in Hugo's diary. He was always so swamped.

The following year, it was my turn to clock fifty. I didn't want a celebration. So instead, I suggested we had a romantic trip on the Orient Express. Hugo booked Paris immediately.

It was a lovely trip. Without the pressure of work, Hugo more than made up for the abstinence in the bedroom. Back home, he further delighted me by presenting me with my new stallion: Zeus. He was absolutely magnificent and wilful. He would be my new adventure.

Zeus needed breaking in, but he thought I would need breaking in too. We were in battle. It was challenging and fun until I got bucked off in the sand school. I was expecting a few tumbles with a new horse. My broken arm was a shock. My previous fracture had been in my childhood. This time it was a more severe break. My pride and spirit were broken too. I was beginning to feel fragile in more ways than one.

The mothers at school mostly expressed concern, a few less so. I overheard:

"It must have been quite a shock for such an excellent horse-woman." "She's always calm and in control; nothing phases her."

"I would be a wreck, very tearful."

"Never mind, it won't be too awkward; she has enough help."

It was true. I had help at home. Nevertheless, the break was inconvenient, more so because it damaged my confidence. I was beginning to feel less sure about everything. The x-ray revealed the beginnings of osteopenia. Was I following in my mother's footsteps after all? Now post-menopausal with the spectre of osteoporosis. Surely not.

Miranda had been marvellous in the fall-out of the broken arm drama. She helped in more ways than I could have anticipated. Yet her main topic of conversation and concern was Hugo. I acknowledged that he looked troubled, but in truth, I was now more irritated at his mood. He had reverted to avoiding intimacy, and I was left craving it again. The Orient Express had just provided a temporary sticking plaster to our *lack-lust-re* existence in the bedroom. In fact, since my fiftieth birthday, my libido was sky high. Yet, my friends were expressing the opposite. I wondered if anything was wrong with me. Was it indeed my libido or was it my need for intimacy?

I knew that, on the surface, I appeared to have it all, but deep down, I felt neglected.

I mourned the loss of my fertile years for a while, reluctantly closing this chapter of wonder and endless possibilities—a time when my self-care was effortless. My hair was glossy, my skin was smooth, my eyes were bright, and I could move with ease. Everything took care of itself back then. The closer I looked, the more I noticed that age was creeping up on me too. My scrutiny is increasingly harsh without my reflection in Hugo's adoring eyes. I was becoming jealous of his cars. When did getting older gain value?

Classic become vintage? I made a mental note to ask Hugo; after all, he gives enough care and attention to his fleet of classic cars. What I've always known, I spent enough time painting them, is that prized cars accentuate feline curves. Their sleek undulations of exaggerated femininity always draw the male gaze. That was my slam-dunk moment; I promised to preserve my femininity at all costs, hoping that desire would follow. In the past, I knew that my aromatherapy baths turned the key with Hugo. Perhaps I could seduce him again if I smelled less like a stable and more like a spa. When I thought my plan was failing, Hugo would surprise me with a night of passion. There was no rhyme or reason, nothing to do with work stress or work success, for that matter. It was just so random

As I was building the courage to have that meaningful but awkward conversation to end my torment, Covid stopped play. Our household all came together and hunkered down. There was nowhere to hide living in such close proximity 24/7. Hugo and I were exposed. He continued to blow hot and cold. My only consolation was that I would know if a mistress existed.

The first twelve weeks were frightening until everyone established personal rhythms. Every household member realised different dreams, engaging in long overdue activities or ones we had procrastinated on. A surge of activity ensued: desks cleared out, spice cupboards reorganised, and the children said farewell to destroyed toys and loose Lego bricks. Everything was online: education, work, shopping, and even social calls with Zoom parties. Let's not forget the scheduled walk a day. All of us were engaged with activities we'd longed to explore with the whole World 'on pause.' Time took on a new dimension; some days felt like snow days, eerie and awfully quiet, and others were full of nature's cacophony: birdsong in the Hampshire countryside, without the hum of traffic, was delightful and deafening.

My emptying nest was full again. My happiness was juxtaposed next to that of Hugo. He was more than worried about the global crisis; he was positively morose. He didn't know how the pandemic would affect his work and our family, and he behaved as if the whole problem was his responsibility. I became irritated with the more he fretted about things outside his control. It was as if he was the sole person withstanding the might of the pandemic with all its consequences. Hugo was gloomy, and we all felt it. I never knew where I stood. I tried to use the family's energy to cheer him up but to little avail. I reclaimed the familiar mantle of mother earth, planting vegetables and cooking up a storm.

No one in the family had caught Covid. We avoided the village, kept ourselves to ourselves, and were primarily self-sufficient anyway. I only appreciated the grim side of the isolation when I went out riding alone one day, and my horse threw me again. Zeus had settled nicely by now, but some fox cubs fell out of the hedge and spooked him. As they diverted, my horse didn't know which way to turn, and I lost my seat. I knew I was broken again. This break in my other arm was nasty. In agony and shaking, battered and bruised, I limped back to the house, and then the whole family had to worry about getting me to the hospital during the pandemic. It was outright misery knowing that a fluke event had caught me out. In the end, a 111 call paved the way to an organised appointment at the fracture clinic in the hospital; my break was clean and would involve a cast, which wasn't funny as it was my painting arm. I felt weak and incapacitated. Hugo was visibly pissed off with the situation. Thank goodness the kids were old enough to help out now that the au-pairs had long since gone. The longer I was immobile, the more I longed to use my right arm, my vibrator arm.

And still, Hugo swerved naked intimacy. Daily I would question, were we at a different stage of our lives? Would we be permanently out of sync, or was it just a new phase of unforeseen and increased anxiety?

I recognised my good fortune and was grateful however, my inner and outer worlds were in flux. This series of events, including the pandemic, made me take stock of my life. Being busy was never my problem. My legacy to our children was always being present and focused on them. As they grew, I would celebrate every milestone. Always mindful of their time to fledge, leaving an empty nest. As each child left for university, it became apparent that I was partly replacing them with a puppy. Our labs had quite a few litters, and we always kept one from each litter. We often say that we're just replacing the heartbeats in the house. The sock-strewn floors continue, how we like it. But the family home was no longer enough. With each year, it was so quickly becoming a museum of past lives. I was feeling levels of loss.

Apart from being a good mother, I needed a new purpose from now on.

Throughout my childhood, my mother was always too busy with various pastimes, especially if they gained validation with accreditations: Reflexology - no clients, Indian head massage - no clients, Pottery - no hardware, Crystallography - no clients. But in truth, all the certificates demonstrated mere distractions with a lack of focus. My father used to describe her self-absorption as "idle-busy."

That will never be me.

My fine arts degree was in the dim and distant past. Yes, I'd dabbled occasionally with small local village exhibitions, nothing serious. My frolicking twenties had been fun, but my various jobs were never intended to result in a career. Over the years, we have bought a bookstore's worth of children's books. Clearing them out lately made me think I could revert my talents to storytelling and painting. I mused that maybe I could write a children's book and illustrate it myself. Whatever my future holds, it would have to have tangible outcomes.

Then out of the blue, a friend, who works for a woman's charity, sent me some photos of women, survivors of breast cancer surgery and asked me to paint portraits to honour their bodies. It was the perfect occupation and project to begin during the lockdowns.

Once life resumed as normal, the commission continued. I was able to go back to my guilty pleasure of life drawing. By painting a series of old and young women, I became visually educated in appreciating the anatomy of humans in all their forms. Feeling almost expert on how the body ages, I noticed that some women's breasts had nipples that pointed to the floor, but others had breasts that just appeared to slide down their ribcage. Of course, all GPs would know that women's breasts have an infinite variety of colours, sizes and shapes. No wonder men find them fascinating. I still like my own with their pretty pink nipples, and so did Hugo, once upon a time.

A surprise this week– a young thirty-something *male,* and he's a *redhead!* He was a true Adonis with a big … ego. Interestingly, he had the same colour, red pubic hair as mine. We noticed each other in the same way breeds of dogs recognise each other. Eye-to-eye contact locked immediately. I found myself admiring his member, which, he clearly knew, was magnificent. I was busy playing with him in my mind while throwing a few flirtatious glances his way. I imagined I could transmit my fantasy of using his apparatus as an ice cream perched on a cone. Daydreaming, I would lick the top, diving my tongue into the soft peak, then licking around the helm, pursing my lips to softly and not so softly kiss the helm, lingering just below the nick of his sweet spot. Then I'd lick the drips along the whole shaft of the cone and return to the peak again. I noticed that his balls were too hairy, oddly, a mismatch with his very groomed head, so I continued my fantasy and smiled. The reclining

Bacchus-like model had caught my train of thought and looked uncomfortable. Was he beginning to inflate? I finished my mental toying by imagining rougher and more urgent mouth and tongue play until he ..." Oh shit!", cold and wet...I'd just caught the brushes in the pot, and the water had spilt all over my crotch.

"Distracted again, India?" said a much older fellow painter.

Another one whispered, "Sourpuss, and I bet she has ..."

"Now, now, be kind," I whispered back. "Solidarity, remember?"

I replied to the question, "Yes, I've got to make a unicorn cake for Maddie's birthday and had some inspiration."

The group quietly tittered.

I discretely changed my focus from his manhood and instead concentrated my efforts on his face. Which, I noticed, was now slightly smirking. I had a crashing realisation, I could have him, but I didn't want him—end of play.

My fantasy in the art class proved that I am still a sexual being, always have been and even now, in my middle years, I still have an appetite. But that's not all. My intimate longing belongs to Hugo. It's always been, Hugo. What I don't know yet is if he, my husband for more than 25 years, longs for me or if it was just a mechanical problem.

I needed to talk to Hugo urgently. If it were a lack of desire, that would be troubling, but if it was the latter, mechanical, it was reassuring and surmountable. But first, I would have to come clean with my discovery of his blue pills. I was recently reminded that intimacy starts with an honest conversation. So I hope we can leave the fears and find the fun again in our love nest.

As suspected, Hugo was about to put his head under the bonnet of his favourite car. "Before you go down on that one, Darling, I have a new game for you. I'll show you my tools if you show me yours." I held out both arms and presented both hands clenched. I said, "Pick a hand." Hugo looked both bemused and perplexed but tapped the left. I turned the hand over and uncurled my fingers to reveal his blue pills, and very quickly opened the other to reveal my pocket vibrator. "Now that we're both equipped, we need to talk."

Amused and relieved by the disclosure, we agreed that that conversation had to wait. Hugo wanted to land his deal first.

So he was spending a couple of nights in town that week. When the hard-fought deal came in, the pressure to perform was immediately replaced by the pressure to celebrate with his young team. A strip club was suggested, and he and his older work, chum, felt obliged to join.

A text message from Hugo. "Success. Pressure off, for now. Off to celebrate. Miss you." It was good that he was missing my tossing with night sweats, but I missed his lump in our bed and the smell of him. I needed him to know that whilst performance at work matters and success is celebrated, success in the bedroom was less to do with performance and more to do with connection. Our tools were mere enablers.

Hugo saw his mobile phone flashing, saw that it was 'home,' and thought: "Shit! First battle won, another awaits." So he let it go to voicemail. Later in the loo, feeling guilty, he picked up the message. According to him, he was smiling like a Cheshire cat as he went back out to join his group.

His old pal and work colleague said, "What's up with you?"

He told the group: "I'm off, chaps. I'm needed at home."

"Anything wrong?" asked his friend.

"No, I think everything is right, by the sound of it," said Hugo quietly. "My wife needs me to share a good bottle of red whilst sharing a bath with her. My kind of threesome, so not likely to be in tomorrow."

"Lucky bastard," said his friend.

He ran for the train, and when seated on board, he listened to my voicemail message again.

*Darling, it's me. Please come home tonight. I need you. Nothing wrong, I just need to tell you three things. Firstly, I love you, always have and always will. Secondly, I like you too, you're my best friend, and that's important. Thirdly, I've been on quite a physical and emotional journey lately. I'm sure you're aware of some of it, but believe me, **you don't know the half of it.** You have a story of your own, I'm sure. So let's cuddle up like old times and talk all night long. Let me know when you're on your way. Then, I'll open a bottle of Margaux, run us a bath, and we can all ... breathe.*

He texted, *ETA 11:36 xxx*

| 14 |

The Wrap-up

Trusted listeners, what a journey this series has been. These media segments have been varied, to say the least: Sometimes whimsical, sometimes dark and heavy, all informative. Along with extensive research, we have married the hard data, fact and figures with your heartfelt submissions. And from your feedback, I'm re-assured that we've covered the topics that really matter to you. My last podcast, apart from a bit of fun, delivered a serious message. In a sense it was a homage to **Everywoman** and the growing need for a sisterhood. As women, we're changing, society is changing and so is the rest of the world. By now you've got to know me and surely I have revealed enough of my life story for you to be assured that I am championing the **Sisterhood**.

The first and last in this series contain tales of feary to fiery queens who have overcome the fears and anxieties of midlife. We leave them as zealous warriors confidently facing their future. You would have spotted by now that these tales are loaded metaphorically and symbolically. These can be as deep as you dare to delve.

So where are we at the end of this series? Let's do a quick recap.

What lies behind the mask?

As women, do we ever reveal all? It's a constant battle of control with the dilemma of what we need to reveal against the harsh exposure that renders us vulnerable. This podcast exposes the myriad of unwelcome menopause symptoms. Even the lack of menstruation doesn't make up for the intrusion of these new ones. Don't you just hate it? Just as we get our act together and start to find the joys in life again, we're side-swiped, thrown off balance. *Hello, menopause.*

Poor Ella. In wanting it all to be over and done with, she was willing to endure hot flushing for 24 hours, the only symptom she associated with menopause. Instead, she learned that she had misjudged the multitude of further symptoms with their different frequencies and intensities. Let's face it; her tale was a ridiculous parody. It was never going to be that extreme in real life.

We will all have a bespoke collection. Ella's tale has taught us that we need to pace ourselves. We need time to adapt. Prepare for the unexpected because sometimes, the transition may even get ridiculous.

We searched and found an available means to track our symptoms because, as we all know, what is playing out today may not be the same tomorrow. It's a simple way to scope - what to tackle and when. And, if there is a need, then involve the professionals. There are always options, medical and otherwise.

Remember, menopause is a moving target.

Let's talk about your privates!

Sex is important. Your 'Privates' matter, and they're undergoing their change too.

Apart from Barry's embarrassment, three listeners offered their questions: the first question was about their libido not matched by their partner and feeling that their sex life was doomed. The second was a concern about their desire for adventurous sex and its consequences as their bits change. The third was an embarrassing admission about incontinence and their fear of further deterioration.

What's the route to finding shared intimacy again? Does the climactic outcome depend on trust-based intimacy, emotional connection, or the basic mechanics? Maybe all of the above with a pinch of fun? In mid-life relationships, who does what? Where are the compromises, and how authentic are any of us prepared to be? As we are laid bare physically whilst being laid bare emotionally. That is the thrust of the matter; communication is everything. When a raging libido is a symptom that cannot be satisfied, it poses risks. There's a risk of temptation, physical and mental distancing. All of which can point to a relationship in crisis - a slippery slope, or not. Either way, now is not the time to avoid awkward conversations.

So let's move on to what adventurous sex in menopause means. We're talking about the mechanics now. If scented candles, dimmed lighting, and soft play are not titillating enough for you, and role-playing dominance or submission is more your predilection, then the only real concern is to lube or not to lube. That certainly is the question. But that just takes care of the locomotion; the bigger concern must surely be. How big a risk are you willing to take to satisfy that thrill? With the dynamic of power-play in mind, who is making the rules, and who is setting the boundaries? It's all a mind game, really.

Pivoting on mechanics and shocking acts, let's address the wet patch on the seat: incontinence. No one wants it, no one likes it, and not many talk about it. But, if you've ever been party to another's distress, you will fear it for yourself. Does this mean you foresee never being without reinforcements or is a medical intervention needed?

With a final flush, when it comes to our privates, take time to have intimate conversations with partners and professionals.

Never give up hope. There are so many OTC products out there. Nothing is inevitable, not even incontinence. There is even more joy to be found here in midlife. No matter what your sexual smorgasbord entails, if you want it, you may yet have the best sex of your life.

Voices in your head

What happens when menopausal symptoms mimic those of mental disorders? Do these symptoms become just added noise - joining the loud chorus of life events and our emotional responses? All of which continue to play out in our heads. Then, layered with day-to-day stressors, is it any wonder we are mistaken for going mad? But times are changing, and we wear our labels now. There is less stigma, we are more informed, so we are taking back control.

Let's explore these voices in this period of tears and fears.

The inner coach is always with us. It chimes in when needed, existing most of the time as an observer. The SELF, inner; unfiltered, and sometimes unfettered; outer, reasoned, and logical. The inner critic needs no introduction – we know this voice too well. Left unchecked, it can so easily dominate. Many have worked out how to silence it, but it can remain the loudest and most damaging inner voice for some. From here, anxiety, depressive thoughts, and panic attacks can surface. All it takes is an unexpected external trigger, like a voice from the past, once dead and buried, now resurfacing. When sustained, the clashing of all the noise can render you impotent. You lose agency. Perhaps now is the time to talk to a professional.

For the rest of us, how do we tune out those voices of caution or amplify those of encouragement to find stability? Balance and perspective are where we find our SELF, the most robust voice. This voice of calm and reasoned certainty knows when to regroup, plan, forge ahead, and navigate our way through periods of distress safely. Whether recovering from a partner's death, changing relationship status, or facing other life-altering decisions, this voice of reason brings back control.

Isn't it about time to conquer your demons, the ghosts from your past that should no longer haunt your present? Once you've unburdened, rejoice in this new lightness, the clarity, and the way forward. Keep asking more questions to understand the interlinking of midlife and menopause. Your future mental health depends on it.

Finally, with this powerful voice, we warn others never to patronise because, as middle-aged women, we don't just get mad; we get … furious.

Ageing and Ageism: Interviews

This decade of healthy ageing is a global initiative from the World Health Organisation and associated parties. And depending on where you are placed around the globe, ageing and ageism are viewed very differently. A blog or a podcast couldn't do this topic justice; instead, I elected for in-depth interviews with three menopausal women and their insights into past, present and future generations and how supported they feel.

As much as our landscape is evolving, our realities are changing, including our perspectives on ageing. As we move from a patriarchal culture into an egalitarian one, the double jeopardy of ageing+female is a growing discussion. So too, are the stigmas around your lifestyle choices and sexual preferences. We're in the twenty-first century, and a slow acceptance is emerging.

Is age revered or feared? That may depend on your circles of influence, from a cultural stance, the legal framework, and any political changes, to local customs and interpretations. All of which informs you – the individual. Perhaps like most, you don't give it much thought until mid-life. Aches and pains give way to illness, which soon becomes a chronic illness, and before you know it, you're invited to be screened for breast, bowel, and cervical irregularities. How supported will you be? It may be time to reframe attitudes.

Studies have indicated that socio-economically placement and geographical location can affect health and longevity—not forgetting individual expectations of happiness. Yet, as we age, the question remains. Will we still have a purpose? With a growing age gap between the young and the old-old, what is needed to keep us contributing to society, to the economy in any shape or form? Is it time to upskill or downscale?

This far into the decade of healthy ageing, are you feeling the sense of urgency yet? Has the rhetoric changed to tangible actions? Change is certainly afoot, but is it happening fast enough? It feels like we will be caught out as we have been with climate change. Decades of chatter, not enough action. Unless *you* plan to safeguard your long-term health and healthcare, you may find your happy and healthy future at risk. The alternative is that you're at the mercy of the State. Depending on how financially equipped and competent it may be. Necessity may mean here come the robot carers, efficient and cost-effective. But studies show that we still need the human touch for longevity.

To find out how change is filtering down to you, let's look at how expansive your community is. Your family, friends, social networks, place of employment, and spiritual connections; are all within the legal, educational, and commercial frameworks. The size of your reach depends on how wide you need it to be. Are you experiencing *anything* associated with this healthy ageing vision?

Or is it just not loud and clear enough?

If Japan has the vision to be the global leader in healthy ageing by 2035, what can we learn from them? Already they have a transparent accountability plan for reporting progress across the levels of self, community, social, and government.

That's part of a much bigger picture; now let's scale this back to you.

In an ideal world, you will have health and mobility, which allows you to move freely without restrictions. With this freedom comes the ability to interact with others, building social networks. With a sense of belonging comes acceptance and a sense of SELF. Contentment follows when all these needs are satisfied. In our modern world, digital interconnectivity is what links it all. Think about it.

Health can be managed with a digital application. So too, can your banking, shopping, home surveillance, transport needs, and so on. Are you still thinking of your device as a help or hindrance? Think again. With the promise that no one should be left behind, how will generations Past, Present, and Future adjust?

What steps have you taken to future-proof the next couple of decades? Remember, it not just about you. Do as much as you can until the rest falls into place.

We concluded this podcast with three important markers that point to success and its associated rewards:

- Control: Change your thinking, feeling, and doing.
- Connect: You are a conduit between the past and future. Safeguard and actively build real-life connections. Understand the role of digital media.
- Health: Look after your health. Live long, live well.

Weathering and Future-proofing: Risk2Reward®

Let's review you and your life's journey so far. How have you weathered? In the game of Risk, think about what is in play for you:

- Lifestyles and habits
- Emotional triggers and your responses
- Genetic predispositions
- Jeopardies
- Family traditions
- Life's events
- Medical history
- Belief systems, religious or otherwise
- Life's stressors (environmental, financial and relationships, and so on)
- Legal, political, social constructs

Are your medical records consistent and up to date? We know that the relevance of prior trauma or conditions, physical or mental, can resurface later in life.

Sustained or momentary, everyone has tripped and fallen at some point. And here we are, in midlife.

You are either *walking tall* or *stumbling and falling* in the game of life. If it's the latter, you have potentially **preloaded health risks** along the way. The time for risk-taking and fast recovery is behind you.

It is knowing that no one is like you and that you are the main agent for change. Are *you* future-proofed yet?

The BTM **Risk2Reward®** model, which incorporates the menopause as an overlay, uncovers your areas (called domains) of imbalance. Whether it be an imbalance in Mind, Body, or Spirit, or across all three, any discrepancies will surface. So it is with *your* input that it reveals the six rewards most relevant to you. Eating, moving, sleeping, being at one with nature, connecting to others - tribe, and finally acceptance of self and others in harmony; are all simple but meaningful rewards. They will be uniquely meaningful to everyone.

This holistic tool, together with the usual standardised health metrics, allow for a bespoke and targeted approach to mapping your healthy future.

After all, it's always best to measure it to manage it. *It's your life.*

The Vanity (Warrior) Project

When it comes to mental, physical, and spiritual health and having actively centred yourself, why are you still wobbling? Good health leads to vitality and an inner glow, so why is that not good enough? It seems as if the beauty standard of this time has its own metrics. Following the rules of old, this template for midlife beauty is … well, rather expensive. These health and beauty ideals should reconcile and not be at odds. We are all participating in this beauty pageant; risks known or unknown, but is it worth the gamble? Whether we do this for comfort, protection or acceptance, or all of the above, the fact is, we do gamble. All the while hoping that the powers that be (the industry and its regulations) have systems in place to safeguard our health. POOF! That's wishful thinking.

Now it's time to call the shots. After all, we pay the price. Queens or not! Start by filtering who you are listening to and influenced by because the starting point is the RAW you, comfortable in your skin—pride overruling vanity.

How far are you willing to go? Next, let's talk layering up. In your world or realm, how many layers will you need to pass muster?

Face: plucked, pampered, painted

Clean: hair, body, teeth

Hair: preened and polished

Pulse points: yep, scented, oops … like an alley cat

Attire: fit for purpose

At which level were you happy in your skin? Or do you feel compelled to take it to the next level of artifice? If you're thinking, that depends; it's all about context. And if you are asking, Where is Wally-mina? The authentic one? The answer is: She's everywhere and she's confident, with or without the mask. Wally-mina has found her sense of pride.

It's time, it's *your* call.

Self-acceptance leads to acceptance by the tribe. A sense of belonging. A tribe that recognises shared principles. The future beauty charter of the Sisterhood, will endorse: transparency, safety, sustainability, and cultural & ethical suitability. Once you appreciate the range and qualities of others, you **stop competing and collaborate instead**. Being part of a tribe that supports each other, you can grow a collective voice, which heralds change—thereby redesigning the blueprint for beauty at any age.

Most importantly, now go and *role-model it!*

In conclusion

If women represent half of the world's population, we are someone's: daughter, sister, mother, or grandmother. We matter. In general, globally, we outlive our men (as the recent pandemic underlined).

That wasn't always the case, but over the last one hundred years, many of us survived the perils of childbirth and no longer die shortly after menopause. So potentially, we have another three decades to live, and we should live them well.

Yes, our bodies and faces will change – that's the privilege of having more years on this beautiful planet. But do we look back with nostalgia to mourn the passing of youth? No, we only review our journey so far to understand our physical and mental preloads. Instead, we can best prepare for the journey ahead by understanding where we are. After all, we want to welcome the future, not fear it.

How do we do that?

As individuals, It's time to control the controllable; we take care of our physical and mental health, keep learning, and ensure that we stay connected.

In our groups, we focus on building our local and global communities. With our collective voices, we call out injustices and call for change. We lobby for good infrastructure and demand regulations protecting our children's future and our own.

As the sandwich generation, we must understand and treasure the past and role model the future.

Imagine what a decade or two ahead could look like.

Wouldn't it be great if our grandchildren, anywhere in the world, when asked, "Where is your happy Granny?" using their devices, check in on us and reply:

- *"It looks like mine is at her poker club"*
- *"Mine is at her work"*
- *"Mine is at the 'teach and learn' intergen hub"*
- *"Mine is out Nordic walking"*
- *"Ok, guys, before you roll your eyes, "mine is out training for the marathon."*

"Well, of course she is; there is always one."

What happy granny will you be?

Notes

What lies behind the mask? (They see/She sees)

1. australian menopause society (2022). *Diagnosing Menopause.* [online] www.menopause.org.au. Available at: http://www.menopause.org.au.
2. org.uk. (2019). *A Guide to Navigating your Menopause.* [online] Available at: A guide to navigating your menopause Bristol Women's Voice https://www.bristolwomensvoice.org.uk › uploads PDF.
3. de Salis, I., Owen-Smith, A., Donovan, J.L. and Lawlor, D.A. (2017). Experiencing menopause in the UK: The interrelated narratives of normality, distress, and transformation. *Journal of Women & Aging*, 30(6), pp.520–540. doi:https://doi.org/10.1080/08952841.2018.1396783.
4. Dinger, J. and Heinemann, L. (n.d.). *Menopause Rating Scale as Outcome Measure for Hormone Treatment.* [online] Available at: https://zeg-berlin.de/wp-content/uploads/2017/01/poster.pdf.
5. Dinger, J., Zimmermann, T., Heinemann, L.A. and Stoehr, D. (2006). Quality of life and hormone use: new validation results of MRS scale. *Health and Quality of Life Outcomes*, 4(1). doi:https://doi.org/10.1186/1477-7525-4-32.
6. Eng, M. (2019). *Estrone Test: High & Low Levels + Normal Range.* [online] SelfDecode Labs. Available at: https://labs.selfdecode.com/blog/estrone-test.
7. Erbil, N. (2015). Menopause attitude, body image and depression of women in menopause. *Maturitas*, 81(1), p.217. doi:https://doi.org/10.1016/j.maturitas.2015.02.339.
8. Erbil, N. (2018). Attitudes towards menopause and depression, body image of women during menopause. *Alexandria Journal of Medicine*, 54(3), pp.241–246. doi:https://doi.org/10.1016/j.ajme.2017.05.012.

9. co.uk. (2015). *oxford health.nhs.uk pain assessment and management*. [online] Available at: https://www.oxfordhealth.nhs.uk/Pain-assessment-tool [Accessed 2021].

10. Harlow, S.D., Gass, M., Hall, J.E., Lobo, R., Maki, P., Rebar, R.W., Sherman, S., Sluss, P.M. and de Villiers, T.J. (2012). Executive Summary of the Stages of Reproductive Aging Workshop + 10: Addressing the Unfinished Agenda of Staging Reproductive Aging. *The Journal of Clinical Endocrinology & Metabolism*, 97(4), pp.1159–1168. doi:https://doi.org/10.1210/jc.2011-3362.

11. Harlow, S.D., Karvonen-Gutierrez, C., Elliott, M.R., Bondarenko, I., Avis, N.E., Bromberger, J.T., Brooks, M.M., Miller, J.M. and Reed, B.D. (2017). It is not just menopause: symptom clustering in the Study of Women's Health Across the Nation. *Women's Midlife Health*, 3(1). doi:https://doi.org/10.1186/s40695-017-0021-y.

12. Heinemann, L.A., DoMinh, T., Strelow, F., Gerbsch, S., Schnitker, J. and Schneider, H.P. (2004a). The Menopause Rating Scale (MRS) as outcome measure for hormone treatment. *Health and Quality of Life Outcomes*, 2(1), p.67. doi:https://doi.org/10.1186/1477-7525-2-67.

13. Heinemann, L.A., DoMinh, T., Strelow, F., Gerbsch, S., Schnitker, J. and Schneider, H.P. (2004b). *Health and Quality of Life Outcomes*, 2(1), p.67. doi:https://doi.org/10.1186/1477-7525-2-67.

14. Heinemann, L.A., Potthoff, P. and Schneider, H.P. (2003). International versions of the Menopause Rating Scale (MRS). *Health and Quality of Life Outcomes*, 1(1), p.28. doi:https://doi.org/10.1186/1477-7525-1-28.

15. Hill, K. (1996). The demography of menopause. *Maturitas*, [online] 23(2), pp.113–127. doi:https://doi.org/10.1016/0378-5122(95)00968-x.

16. Marshall, L. (2015). Menopause. *Nature Reviews Disease Primers*, 1(1). doi:https://doi.org/10.1038/nrdp.2015.54.

17. National Library of Medicine (2022). *A menopause-specific quality of life questionnaire National Institutes of Health (.gov) https://pubmed.ncbi.nlm.nih.gov › ... by JR Hilditch · 1996 · Cited by 778 — The MENQOL (Menopause-Specific Quality*. [online] PubMed. Available at: https://pubmed.ncbi.nlm.nih.gov.

18. NCC-WCH Version 1.2 Menopause Appendices A - G Clinical Guideline Methods, evidence and recommendations 1 June 2015 Commissioned by the National Institute for Health and Clinical Excellence Draft for Consultation. (2015).

19. NIH Office of Dietary Supplements 08/05/2019 Black Cohosh — Health Professional Fact Sheet Black Cohosh. (2018). [online] od.nih.gov. Available at: http://ods.od.nih.gov/factsheets/BlackCohosh-HealthProfessiona/5098/hist.

20. Radtke, J.V. (2011). *The Menopause-Specific Quality of Life (MEN-QOL)*. [online] National Institute of Heath. Available at: https://www.ncbi.nlm.nih.gov [Accessed 2021].

21. Research on the menopause in the 1990s. Report of a WHO Scientific Group. (1996). *Research on the menopause in the 1990's*, 866(1996 Vol 866), pp.1–107.

22. Santoro, N. and Sutton-Tyrrell, K. (2011). The SWAN Song: Study of Women's Health Across the Nation's Recurring Themes. *Obstetrics and Gynecology Clinics of North America*, 38(3), pp.417–423. doi:https://doi.org/10.1016/j.ogc.2011.05.001.

23. Schneider, H.P.G., Heinemann, L.A.J., Rosemeier, H.-P. ., Potthoff, P. and Behre, H.M. (2000). The Menopause Rating Scale (MRS): comparison with Kupperman index and quality-of-life scale SF-36. *Climacteric*, 3(1), pp.50–58. doi:https://doi.org/10.3109/13697130009167599.

24. Services, D. of H. & H. (n.d.). *Premature and early menopause.* [online] www.betterhealth.vic.gov.au. Available at: https://www.betterhealth.vic.gov.au/health/conditionsandtreatments/premature-and-early-menopause.

25. (2021). *SheCares - Women's Health and Hormonal Imbalance premature menopause.* [online] Available at: https://www.shecares.com [Accessed Feb. 2021].

26. Wallace, D.L. (2011). Literary portrayals of ageing. *Cambridge University Press eBooks*, pp.389–415. doi:https://doi.org/10.1017/cbo9780511973697.014

Let's talk about your privates

1. Age UK. (n.d.). *Sex in later life / Health and wellbeing.* [online] Available at: https://www.ageuk.org.uk/northern-ireland/information-advice/health-wellbeing/relationships-family/sex-in-later-life/.

2. Christofides, A., Swallow, T. and Parkinson, R. (2013). Contemporary Management of recurrent UTI in adult females. *Journal of Clinical Urology*, 6(3), pp.140–147. doi:https://doi.org/10.1177/2051415812472433.

3. Dalrymple, J. (2016). *Why Over 45s are at Risk of Sexually Transmitted Infections.* [online] The Conversation. Available at: https://www.theconversation.com.

4. Hogg, E., Frank, S., Oft, J., Benway, B., Rashid, M.H. and Lahiri, S. (2022). Urinary Tract Infection in Parkinson's Disease. *Journal of Parkinson's Disease*, 12(3), pp.743–757. doi:https://doi.org/10.3233/jpd-213103.

5. Martinez, K. (2017). BDSM Role Fluidity: A Mixed-Methods Approach to Investigating Switches Within Dominant/Submissive Binaries. *Journal of Homosexuality*, 65(10), pp.1299–1324. doi:https://doi.org/10.1080/00918369.2017.1374062.

6. Nappi, R.E., Albani, F., Santamaria, V., Tonani, S., Magri, F., Martini, E., Chiovato, L. and Polatti, F. (2010). Hormonal and psycho-relational aspects of sexual function during menopausal transition and at early menopause. *Maturitas*, [online] 67(1), pp.78–83. doi:https://doi.org/10.1016/j.maturitas.2010.05.008.

7. NHS (2017). *Vaginal dryness.* [online] nhs.uk. Available at: https://www.nhs.uk/conditions/vaginal-dryness/.

8. Sion, S. (2017). *Yes, you can have better sex in midlife and in the years beyond.* [online] Harvard Health. Available at: https://www.health.harvard.edu/womens-health/yes-you-can-have-better-sex-in-midlife-and-in-the-years-beyond.

9. Stephens, C. (2019). *Why Orgasmic Meditation May be the Relaxing Technique You Need.* [online] Healthline. Available at: https://www.healthline.com>orgasmicmeditation-101.

Voices in your head

1. Angermeyer, M.C. and Dietrich, S. (2006). Public beliefs about and attitudes towards people with mental illness: a review of population studies. *Acta Psychiatrica Scandinavica*, 113(3), pp.163–179.

2. Antoniou, E., Rigas, N., Orovou, E., Papatrechas, A. and Sarella, A. (2021). ADHD Symptoms in Females of Childhood, Adolescent, Reproductive and Menopause Period. *Materia Socio Medica*, 33(2), p.114. doi:https://doi.org/10.5455/msm.2021.33.114-118.

3. González-Rodríguez, A. and Seeman, M.V. (2019). The association between hormones and antipsychotic use: a focus on postpartum

and menopausal women. *Therapeutic Advances in Psychopharmacology*, 9, p.204512531985997. doi:https://doi.org/10.1177/2045125319859973.

4. Gordon, J.L., Peltier, A., Grummisch, J.A. and Sykes Tottenham, L. (2019). Estradiol Fluctuation, Sensitivity to Stress, and Depressive Symptoms in the Menopause Transition: A Pilot Study. *Frontiers in Psychology*, 10. doi:https://doi.org/10.3389/fpsyg.2019.01319.

5. Health and Safety Executive. (2021). *Work-related stress, anxiety or depression in Great Britain*. [online] Available at: https://press.hse.gov.uk>2022/11/23>she-publishers.

6. Heinemann, L.A., DoMinh, T., Strelow, F., Gerbsch, S., Schnitker, J. and Schneider, H.P. (2004). *Health and Quality of Life Outcomes*, 2(1), p.67. doi:https://doi.org/10.1186/1477-7525-2-67.

7. Henry, E. and Hill Jones, S. (2011). Experiences of Older Adult Women Diagnosed with Attention Deficit Hyperactivity Disorder. *Journal of Women & Aging*, 23(3), pp.246–262. doi:https://doi.org/10.1080/08952841.2011.589285.

8. House of Commons Women and Equalities Committee Menopause and the workplace survey results Fourth Special Report of Session 2021–22 Ordered by the House of Commons to be printed 23 February 2022. (n.d.).

9. Iacoviello, B.M. and Charney, D.S. (2014). Psychosocial facets of resilience: implications for preventing posttrauma psychopathology, treating trauma survivors, and enhancing community resilience. *European Journal of Psychotraumatology*, 5(1), p.23970. doi:https://doi.org/10.3402/ejpt.v5.23970.

10. Integral Care. (n.d.). *8 Simples Steps to Improve Happiness*. [online] Available at: https://integralcare.org/en/8-simples-steps-to-improve-happiness/.

11. Kirkbride, J.B., Errazuriz, A., Croudace, T.J., Morgan, C., Jackson, D., Boydell, J., Murray, R.M. and Jones, P.B. (2012). Incidence of Schizophrenia and Other Psychoses in England, 1950–2009: A Systematic Review and Meta-Analyses. *PLoS ONE*, 7(3), p.e31660. doi:https://doi.org/10.1371/journal.pone.0031660.

12. McManus, S., Bebbington, P.E., Jenkins, R. and Brugha, T. (2016). *Mental Health and Wellbeing in England: the Adult Psychiatric Morbidity Survey 2014*. [online] openaccess.city.ac.uk. Available at: https://openaccess.city.ac.uk/id/eprint/23646/.

13. NHS (2016). *Adult Psychiatric Morbidity Survey: Survey of Mental Health and Wellbeing, England, 2014 - NHS Digital*. [online] NHS Digital. Available

at: https://digital.nhs.uk/data-and-information/publications/statistical/adult-psychiatric-morbidity-survey/adult-psychiatric-morbidity-survey-survey-of-mental-health-and-wellbeing-england-2014.

14. NHS (2021a). *Feelings and symptoms.* [online] nhs.uk. Available at: https://www.nhs.uk/mental-health/feelings-symptoms-behaviours/feelings-and-symptoms/.

15. NHS (2021b). *Mental Health Services.* [online] nhs.uk. Available at: https://www.nhs.uk/nhs-services/mental-health-services/.

16. NHS Digital. (n.d.). *Adult Psychiatric Morbidity Survey: Survey of Mental Health and Wellbeing, England, 2014.*[online] Available at: https://digital.nhs.uk/catalogue/PUB21748.

17. Public health England (2020). *Prescribed Medicines Review: Summary.* [online] GOV.UK. Available at: https://www.gov.uk/government/publications/prescribed-medicines-review-report/prescribed-medicines-review-summary.

18. Pushkin Industries. (n.d.). *The Happiness Lab with Dr. Laurie Santos.* [online] Available at: https://www.pushkin.fm/podcasts/the-happiness-lab-with-dr-laurie-santos.

19. Szeliga, A., Stefanowski, B., Meczekalski, B., Snopek, M., Kostrzak, A., Smolarczyk, R., Bala, G., Duszewska, A., Smolarczyk, K. and Maciejewska-Jeske, M. (2021). Menopause in women with schizophrenia, schizoaffective disorder and bipolar disorder. *Maturitas*, 152, pp.57–62. doi:https://doi.org/10.1016/j.maturitas.2021.07.003.

20. Velligan, D., Prihoda, T., Dennehy, E., Biggs, M., Shores-Wilson, K., Crismon, M.L., Rush, A.J., Miller, A., Suppes, T., Trivedi, M., Kashner, T.M., Witte, B., Toprac, M., Carmody, T., Chiles, J. and Shon, S. (2005). Brief Psychiatric Rating Scale Expanded Version: How do new items affect factor structure? *Psychiatry Research*, 135(3), pp.217–228. doi:https://doi.org/10.1016/j.psychres.2005.05.001.

21. Warwick Medical School (2017). *The Warwick-Edinburgh Mental Wellbeing Scale (WEMWBS).* [online] Warwick.ac.uk. Available at: https://warwick.ac.uk/fac/sci/med/research/platform/wemwbs/.

22. Watson, S. (2021). *Anxiety & Stress Disorders.* [online] *Google Books.* Harvard Health Publishing. Available at: https://books.google.co.uk/books/about/Anxiety_Stress_Disorders.html?id=jYWbzgEACAAJ&redir_esc=y.

Ageing and Ageism: Interviews in the West, East and somewhere in between

1. Age UK (2018). *Our Research | Age UK*. [online] Ageuk.org.uk. Available at: https://www.ageuk.org.uk/our-impact/policy-research/.
2. Age UK (2019). *Policy positions | Age UK*. [online] Ageuk.org.uk. Available at: https://www.ageuk.org.uk/our-impact/policy-research/policy-positions/.
3. ageing-better.org.uk. (n.d.). *Reframing ageing: Public perceptions of ageing, older age and demographic change | Centre for Ageing Better*. [online] Available at: https://ageing-better.org.uk/resources/reframing-ageing-public-perceptions-ageing-older-age-and-demographic-change.
4. Bahl, N.K.H., Nafstad, H.E., Blakar, R.M. and Geirdal, A.Ø. (2017). Responsibility for Psychological Sense of Community and Well-Being in Old Age: A Qualitative Study of Urban Older Adults in Norway. *Open Journal of Social Sciences*, 05(07), pp.321–338. doi:https://doi.org/10.4236/jss.2017.57020.
5. Berger, R. (2017). Aging in America: Ageism and General Attitudes toward Growing Old and the Elderly. *Open Journal of Social Sciences*, [online] 05(08), pp.183–198. doi:https://doi.org/10.4236/jss.2017.58015.
6. BOUDINY, K. (2012). 'Active ageing': from empty rhetoric to effective policy tool. *Ageing and Society*, 33(6), pp.1077–1098. doi:https://doi.org/10.1017/s0144686x1200030x.
7. Centre for Ageing Better (2022). *Summary | The State of Ageing 2022 | Centre for Ageing Better*. [online] ageing-better.org.uk. Available at: https://ageing-better.org.uk/summary-state-ageing-2022.
8. cycles, T. text provides general information S. assumes no liability for the information given being complete or correct D. to varying update and Text, S.C.D.M. up-to-Date D.T.R. in the (n.d.). *Topic: Social media and children in the UK*. [online] Statista. Available at: https://www.statista.com/topics/9445/social-media-and-children-in-the-uk/#editorsPicks.
9. Harlow, S.D., Burnett-Bowie, S.-A.M., Greendale, G.A., Avis, N.E., Reeves, A.N., Richards, T.R. and Lewis, T.T. (2022). Disparities in Reproductive Aging and Midlife Health between Black and White women: The Study of Women's Health Across the Nation (SWAN). *Women's Midlife Health*, 8(1). doi:https://doi.org/10.1186/s40695-022-00073-y.

10. Hill, K. (n.d.). *The demography of menopause.*

11. Home & Community: The Ageing Tsunami Introduction: the nature of 'home'. (2013).

12. Hvas, L. (2006). Menopausal women's positive experience of growing older. *Maturitas*, 54(3), pp.245–251. doi:https://doi.org/10.1016/j.maturitas.2005.11.006.

13. Kalfoss, M. (2016). Gender Differences in Attitudes to Ageing among Norwegian Older Adults. *Open Journal of Nursing*, 06(03), pp.255–266. doi:https://doi.org/10.4236/ojn.2016.63026.

14. Kelly, J. (n.d.). *The 'Sandwich Generation' Is Financially Taking Care Of Their Parents, Kids And Themselves.* [online] Forbes. Available at: https://www.forbes.com/sites/jackkelly/2023/02/24/the-sandwich-generation-is-financially-taking-care-of-their-parents-kids-and-themselves/?sh=fccc6b72af4c.

15. Lord Hodgson of Astley Abbotts Britain's Demographic Challenge. (n.d.). Available at: https://www.civitas.org.uk/content/files/britainsdemographicchallengeweb.pdf.

16. Merz, B. (2010). *A Guide to Women's Health.* Harvard Health Publications.

17. Morgan, L. (n.d.). • Allostatic Load: everything you need to know about the stress condition/Glamour Uk – Morgan,Lucy.

18. Nations, U. (2019a). *World Population Ageing 2019 Highlights.* United Nations.

19. Organization, W.H. (2018). *Global action plan on physical activity 2018–2030: more active people for a healthier world.* [online] who.int. World Health Organization. Available at: https://apps.who.int/iris/handle/10665/272722.

20. Parker, K. and Patten, E. (2013). *The sandwich generation.* [online] Pew Research Center's Social & Demographic Trends Project. Available at: https://www.pewresearch.org/social-trends/2013/01/30/the-sandwich-generation/.

21. Policy Position Paper Ageism and Age Equality. (2020). Available at: https://www.ageuk.org.uk/globalassets/age-uk/documents/policy-positions/cross-cutting-issues/ageism-and-age-equality-feb-2020.pdf.

22. PRB (2018). *Population Reference Bureau – Inform, Empower, Advance.* [online] Prb.org. Available at: https://www.prb.org/.

23. Schoenaker, D.A., Jackson, C.A., Rowlands, J.V. and Mishra, G.D. (2014). Socioeconomic position, lifestyle factors and age at natural menopause: a systematic review and meta-analyses of studies across six

continents. *International Journal of Epidemiology*, [online] 43(5), pp.1542–1562. doi:https://doi.org/10.1093/ije/dyu094.

24. Smith, P.K. (2008). Cyberbullying: its nature and impact in secondary school pupils. *Journal of child psychology and psychiatry, and allied disciplines*, [online] 49(4), pp.376–85. doi:https://doi.org/10.1111/j.1469-7610.2007.01846.x.

25. Steptoe, A. and Zaninotto, P. (2020). Lower socioeconomic status and the acceleration of aging: An outcome-wide analysis. *Proceedings of the National Academy of Sciences*, 117(26), pp.14911–14917. doi:https://doi.org/10.1073/pnas.1915741117.

26. Tuohy, D. and Cooney, A. (2019). Older Women's Experiences of Aging and Health: An Interpretive Phenomenological Study. *Gerontology and Geriatric Medicine*, [online] 5, p.233372141983430. doi:https://doi.org/10.1177/2333721419834308.

27. United Nations (2019b). *World population prospects 2019*. [online] United Nations. Available at: https://population.un.org/wpp/Publications/Files/WPP2019_Highlights.pdf.

28. United Nations (2022). *World population prospects - population division - united nations*. [online] UN. Available at: https://population.un.org/wpp/.

29. van den Eijnden, R.J.J.M., Lemmens, J.S. and Valkenburg, P.M. (2016). The Social Media Disorder Scale. *Computers in Human Behavior*, [online] 61(61), pp.478–487. doi:https://doi.org/10.1016/j.chb.2016.03.038.

30. H.O. (2021). *Ageing and health*. [online] www.who.int. Available at: https://who.int/news-room/fact-sheets/detail/ageing-and-health.

31. WALKER, A. (2017). Why the UK Needs a Social Policy on Ageing. *Journal of Social Policy*, 47(2), pp.253–273. doi:https://doi.org/10.1017/s0047279417000320.

32. Williams, D.R. and Purdie-Vaughns, V. (2016). Needed Interventions to Reduce Racial/Ethnic Disparities in Health: Table 1. *Journal of Health Politics, Policy and Law*, 41(4), pp.627–651. doi:https://doi.org/10.1215/03616878-3620857.

33. World Economic Forum (2020). *Global Gender Gap Report 2020*. [online] Available at: https://www3.weforum.org/docs/WEF_GGGR_2020.pdf.

34. World Health Organisation (2021). *Coronavirus disease (COVID-19)*. [online] World Health Organization. Available at: https://www.who.int/health-topics/coronavirus#tab=tab_1.

35. housinglin.org.uk. (2013). *Home and Community: An ageing tsunami*. [on-line] Available at: https://www.housinglin.org.uk/Topics/type/Home-and-Community-An-ageing-tsunami/.
36. who.int. (n.d.). *Decade of Healthy Ageing (2021-2030)*. [on-line] Available at: https://www.who.int/initiatives/decade-of-healthy-ageing#:~:text=The%20United%20Nations%20Decade%20of.

Interviews - the West

1. *"The Economic Status of Women in West Virginia" Fact Sheet IWPR #R529, March 2018*. Mar. 2018, www.statusofwomendata.org.
2. Alegría, Margarita, et al. "Disparity in Depression Treatment among Racial and Ethnic Minority Populations in the United States." *Psychiatric Services*, vol. 59, no. 11, Nov. 2008, pp. 1264–1272, https://doi.org/10.1176/ps.2008.59.11.1264.
3. Avenue, Next. "America's Best and Worst States to Grow Old." *Forbes*, www.forbes.com/sites/nextavenue/2017/08/17/americas-best-and-worst-states-to-grow-old/?sh=96c75748f698.
4. Bell, Jennifer. *Boost Your New Year with These Healthy Dining Options - Visit Harrisonburg Virginia in the Shenandoah Valley*. 22 Dec. 2021, www.visitharrisonburgva.com/boost-your-new-year-healthy-dining/.
5. de la Fuente, Javier, et al. "Are Younger Cohorts in the USA and England Ageing Better?" *International Journal of Epidemiology*, vol. 48, no. 6, 25 June 2019, pp. 1906–1913, https://doi.org/10.1093/ije/dyz126.
6. "Explore Obesity - Women in West Virginia | AHR." *America's Health Rankings*, www.americashealthrankings.org/explore/measures/Obesity_women/WV.
7. "Explore Overall in West Virginia | AHR." *America's Health Rankings*, www.americashealthrankings.org/explore/measures/Overall/WV.
8. "Growing Old in West Virginia - the Good, the Bad and the Ugly." *HuffPost*, 10 June 2010, www.huffpost.com/entry/growing-old-in-west-virgi_b_607969.
9. "ISPOR - US Healthcare System Overview-Backgound." *Www.ispor.org*, 2022, www.ispor.org/heor-resources/more-heor-resources/us-health-

care-system-overview/us-healthcare-system-overview-background-page-1.

10. Law, Colombo. "Unbelievable Car Accident Statistics in West Virginia." *Colombo Law*, 9 Aug. 2018, www.colombolaw.com/west-virginia-blog/west-virginia-car-accident-statistics/.

11. Lu, Wentian, et al. "Comparing Socio-Economic Inequalities in Healthy Ageing in the United States of America, England, China and Japan: Evidence from Four Longitudinal Studies of Ageing." *Ageing and Society*, 9 Dec. 2019, pp. 1–26, https://doi.org/10.1017/s0144686x19001740.

12. Magazine, Smithsonian. "Buckhannon, West Virginia: The Perfect Birthplace." *Smithsonian Magazine*, www.smithsonianmag.com/travel/buckhannon-west-virginia-the-perfect-birthplace-11723859/.

13. Mather, Mark, et al. *Ageing in the United States.*

14. ---. "Fact Sheet: Aging in the United States." *Population Reference Bureau*, 15 July 2019, www.prb.org/resources/fact-sheet-aging-in-the-united-states/.

15. Mather, Mark , and Lillian Kilduff. "The U.S. Population Is Growing Older, and the Gender Gap in Life Expectancy Is Narrowing." *PRB*, 19 Feb. 2020, www.prb.org/resources/u-s-population-is-growing-older/.

16. MIT Medical. "Healthcare in the United States: The Top Five Things You Need to Know | MIT Medical." *edu*, MIT Medical, 2019, medical.mit.edu/my-mit/internationals/healthcare-united-states.

17. NW, 1615 L. St, et al. "Growing Old in America: Expectations vs. Reality." *Pew Research Center's Social & Demographic Trends Project*, 29 June 2009, www.pewresearch.org/social-trends/2009/06/29/growing-old-in-america-expectations-vs-reality/.

18. "Silver Tsunami Is Coming to Healthcare: Time to Prepare." *Healthcare IT News*, 15 Mar. 2019, www.healthcareitnews.com/news/silver-tsunami-coming-healthcare-time-prepare.

19. "Stats of the State of West Virginia." *cdc.gov*, 24 May 2019, www.cdc.gov/nchs/pressroom/states/westvirginia/westvirginia.htm.

20. Taylor, Paul, and Kim Parker. *The Sandwich Generation Rising Financial Burdens for Middle-Aged Americans Social & Demographic Trends.* 2013.

21. "The 9 Best Diners in West Virginia!" *com*, bestthingswv.com/diners/#gsc.tab=0.

22. "The West Virginia Senior Living Directory." *org*, www.seniorliving.org/west-virginia/.

23. Thomas, Annette Joan, et al. "The Challenges of Midlife Women: Themes from the Seattle Midlife Women's Health Study." *Women's Midlife Health*, vol. 4, no. 1, 15 June 2018, https://doi.org/10.1186/s40695-018-0039-9.
24. "Women's Leadership Initiative | Home." *wvu.edu*, womensleadership.wvu.edu.

Interviews - the East

1. Airth, Johanna. "What the Japanese Can Teach Us about Super-Ageing Gracefully." *bbc.com*, 30 Mar. 2020, www.bbc.com/future/article/20200327-what-the-japanese-can-teach-about-super-ageing-gracefully.
2. *AT a GLANCE Scientific Foresight: What If?*
3. Ayalon, Liat, and Senjooti Roy. "Combatting Ageism in the Western Pacific Region." *The Lancet Regional Health - Western Pacific*, vol. 35, June 2023, p. 100593, https://doi.org/10.1016/j.lanwpc.2022.100593.
4. D'Ambrogio, Enrico. *Japan's Ageing Society*. Dec. 2020.
5. Dicker, Daniel, et al. "Global, Regional, and National Age-Sex-Specific Mortality and Life Expectancy, 1950–2017: A Systematic Analysis for the Global Burden of Disease Study 2017." *The Lancet*, vol. 392, no. 10159, Nov. 2018, pp. 1684–1735, www.sciencedirect.com/science/article/pii/S0140673618318919, https://doi.org/10.1016/s0140-6736(18)31891-9.
6. "Health Japan 21." *nibiohn.go.jp*, www.nibiohn.go.jp/eiken/kenkounippon21/en/.
7. Ishii, Shinya, et al. "The State of Health in Older Adults in Japan: Trends in Disability, Chronic Medical Conditions and Mortality." *PLOS ONE*, vol. 10, no. 10, 2 Oct. 2015, p. e0139639, https://doi.org/10.1371/journal.pone.0139639.
8. Kincaid, Chris. "A Look at Gender Expectations in Japanese Society." *Japan Powered*, Japan Powered, 8 July 2013, www.japanpowered.com/japan-culture/a-look-at-gender-expectations-in-japanese-society.
9. ---. "Gender Roles of Women in Modern Japan." *Japan Powered*, Japan Powered, 22 June 2014, www.japanpowered.com/japan-culture/gender-roles-women-modern-japan.
10. *Leading the World through Health Provisional Translation.*

11. Nojiri, Shuko, et al. "Comorbidity Status in Hospitalized Elderly in Japan: Analysis from National Database of Health Insurance Claims and Specific Health Checkups." *Scientific Reports*, vol. 9, no. 1, Dec. 2019, https://doi.org/10.1038/s41598-019-56534-4.

12. Nomura, Shuhei, et al. "Toward a Third Term of Health Japan 21 – Implications from the Rise in Non-Communicable Disease Burden and Highly Preventable Risk Factors." *The Lancet Regional Health - Western Pacific*, vol. 21, 1 Apr. 2022, p. 100377, www.sciencedirect.com/science/article/pii/S2666606521002868, https://doi.org/10.1016/j.lanwpc.2021.100377.

13. Publishing, Harvard Health. "What Does It Take to Be a Super-Ager?" *Harvard Health*, www.health.harvard.edu/healthy-aging/what-does-it-take-to-be-a-super-ager.

14. Sudo, Kyoko, et al. "Japan's Healthcare Policy for the Elderly through the Concepts of Self-Help (Ji-Jo), Mutual Aid (Go-Jo), Social Solidarity Care (Kyo-Jo), and Governmental Care (Ko-Jo)." *BioScience Trends*, vol. 12, no. 1, 2018, pp. 7–11, www.jstage.jst.go.jp/article/bst/12/1/12_2017.01271/_pdf/-char/ja, https://doi.org/10.5582/bst.2017.01271.

15. Swain, Frank. "The Technologies That Could Transform Ageing." *bbc.com*, www.bbc.com/future/article/20201104-the-technologies-that-could-transform-ageing#:~:text=A%20tech%2Dempowered%20workforce%2C%20trained.

16. Vauclair, Christin-Melanie, et al. "Are Asian Cultures Really Less Ageist than Western Ones? It Depends on the Questions Asked." *International Journal of Psychology*, vol. 52, no. 2, 4 July 2016, pp. 136–144, www.ncbi.nlm.nih.gov/pmc/articles/PMC5347948/, https://doi.org/10.1002/ijop.12292.

Weathering and Future-proofing. Risk to Reward (part 1)

1. Alebna, P. and Maleki, N. (2021). Allostatic Load in Perimenopausal Women With Migraine. *Frontiers in Neurology*, 12. doi:https://doi.org/10.3389/fneur.2021.649423.

2. American Psychological Association (2021). *Fact sheet: Health disparities and stress.* [online] Apa.org. Available at: https://www.apa.org/topics/racism-bias-discrimination/health-disparities-stress.

3. An, S., Ji, L.-J., Marks, M. and Zhang, Z. (2017). Two Sides of Emotion: Exploring Positivity and Negativity in Six Basic Emotions across Cultures. *Frontiers in Psychology*, 8. doi:https://doi.org/10.3389/fpsyg.2017.00610.

4. org. (2021). Available at: https://www.apa.org/topics/racism-bias-discrimination/health-disparities-stress.pdf.

5. Aspray, T.J. and Hill, T.R. (2019). Osteoporosis and the Ageing Skeleton. *Subcellular Biochemistry*, 91, pp.453–476. doi:https://doi.org/10.1007/978-981-13-3681-2_16.

6. Best To Not Sweat The Small Stuff, Because It Could Kill You. (n.d.). *org*. [online] Available at: https://www.npr.org/sections/health-shots/2014/09/22/349875448/best-to-not-sweat-the-small-stuff-because-it-could-kill-you#:~:text=Chronic%20stress%20is%20hazardous%20to.

7. British Heart Foundation (2023). *Our vision is a world free from the fear of heart and circulatory diseases. UK Factsheet.* [online] Available at: https://www.bhf.org.uk/-/media/files/for-professionals/research/heart-statistics/bhf-cvd-statistics-uk-factsheet.pdf.

8. British Heart Foundation. (n.d.). *Physical inactivity.* [online] Available at: https://www.bhf.org.uk/informationsupport/risk-factors/physical-inactivity#:~:text=How%20active%20do%20I%20need.

9. Collins, S.V. and Hines, A.L. (2021). Stress Reduction to Decrease Hypertension for Black Women: A Scoping Review of Trials and Interventions. *Journal of Racial and Ethnic Health Disparities*. doi:https://doi.org/10.1007/s40615-021-01160-y.

10. Daly, E., Gray, A., Barlow, D., McPherson, K., Roche, M. and Vessey, M. (1993). Measuring the impact of menopausal symptoms on quality of life. *BMJ*, 307(6908), pp.836–840. doi:https://doi.org/10.1136/bmj.307.6908.836.

11. de Salis, I., Owen-Smith, A., Donovan, J.L. and Lawlor, D.A. (2017). Experiencing menopause in the UK: The interrelated narratives of normality, distress, and transformation. *Journal of Women & Aging*, 30(6), pp.520–540. doi:https://doi.org/10.1080/08952841.2018.1396783.

12. Douglas-Cowie, E., Cox, C., Martin, J.-C., Devillers, L., Cowie, R., Sneddon, I.N., McRorie, M., Pelachaud, C., Peters, C.L., Lowry, O.M., Batliner, A. and Florian Hönig (2010). The HUMAINE Database. pp.243–284. doi:https://doi.org/10.1007/978-3-642-15184-2_14.

13. Editor (2019). *The waist to hip ratio calculator gives determines the possibility of health risks and is an indication of whether you have an apple or pear shaped*

figure.[online] Diabetes. Available at: https://www.diabetes.co.uk/waist-to-hip-ratio-calculator.html.

14. Geronimus, A.T. (1992). THE WEATHERING HYPOTHESIS AND THE HEALTH OF AFRICAN-AMERICAN WOMEN AND INFANTS: EVIDENCE AND SPECULATIONS. *Ethnicity & Disease*, [online] 2(3), pp.207–221. Available at: https://www.jstor.org/stable/45403051.

15. UK. (n.d.). *Chief Medical Officer's annual report 2020: health trends and variation in England.* [online] Available at: https://www.gov.uk/government/publications/chief-medical-officers-annual-report-2020-health-trends-and-variation-in-england.

16. Goymann, W. and Wingfield, J.C. (2004). Allostatic load, social status and stress hormones: the costs of social status matter. *Animal Behaviour*, 67(3), pp.591–602. doi:https://doi.org/10.1016/j.anbehav.2003.08.007.

17. Gupta, S. (2006). Obesity and female hormones. *The Obstetrician & Gynaecologist*, 8(1), pp.26–31. doi:https://doi.org/10.1576/toag.8.1.026.27205.

18. Hagey, A.R. and Warren, M.P. (2008). Role of Exercise and Nutrition in Menopause. *Clinical Obstetrics and Gynecology*, [online] 51(3), pp.627–641. doi:https://doi.org/10.1097/GRF.0b013e318180ba84.

19. Hidalgo-Mora, J.J., Cortés-Sierra, L., García-Pérez, M.-Á., Tarín, J.J. and Cano, A. (2020). Diet to Reduce the Metabolic Syndrome Associated with Menopause. The Logic for Olive Oil. *Nutrients*, 12(10), p.3184. doi:https://doi.org/10.3390/nu12103184.

20. Houston, E. (2019). *4 Positive Psychology Exercises To Do With Clients or Students.* [online] PositivePsychology.com. Available at: https://positivepsychology.com/positive-psychology-exercises/.

21. Humphreys, S. (2010). The Unethical Use of BMI in Contemporary General Practice. *British Journal of General Practice*, [online] 60(578), pp.696–697. doi:https://doi.org/10.3399/bjgp10x515548.

22. Iacoviello, B.M. and Charney, D.S. (2014). Psychosocial facets of resilience: implications for preventing posttrauma psychopathology, treating trauma survivors, and enhancing community resilience. *European Journal of Psychotraumatology*, 5(1), p.23970. doi:https://doi.org/10.3402/ejpt.v5.23970.

23. Integral Care. (n.d.). *8 Simples Steps to Improve Happiness.* [online] Available at: https://integralcare.org/en/8-simples-steps-to-improve-happiness/.

24. John Hopkins Medicine (2019) *The Science of Sleep: Understanding What Happens When You Sleep.* [online] Johns Hopkins Medicine Health Library.

Available at: https://www.hopkinsmedicine.org/health/wellness-and-prevention/the-science-of-sleep-understanding-what-happens-when-you-sleep.

25. Lay Summary Ethnic and socio-economic inequalities in NHS maternity and perinatal care for women and their babies. (n.d.). Available at: https://maternityaudit.org.uk/FilesUploaded/RCOG_Inequalities%20Report_Lay_Summary.pdf.

26. Lee, D. (2000). An analysis of workplace bullying in the UK. *Personnel Review*, 29(5), pp.593–610. doi:https://doi.org/10.1108/00483480010296410.

27. Lindsay, R. (2004). Hormones and Bone Health in Postmenopausal Women. *Endocrine*, 24(3), pp.223–230. doi:https://doi.org/10.1385/endo:24:3:223.

28. Mind (2021). *How Nature Benefits Mental Health*. [online] www.mind.org.uk. Available at: https://www.mind.org.uk/information-support/tips-for-everyday-living/nature-and-mental-health/how-nature-benefits-mental-health/.

29. Povoroznyuk, V., Dzerovych, N. and Povoroznyuk, R. (2016). The role of vitamin D and exercises in correction of age-related skeletal muscle changes in postmenopausal women. *Bone Abstracts*. doi:https://doi.org/10.1530/boneabs.5.p262.

30. Public Health England (2018). *Chapter 3: trends in morbidity and risk factors*. [online] GOV.UK. Available at: https://www.gov.uk/government/publications/health-profile-for-england-2018/chapter-3-trends-in-morbidity-and-risk-factors.

31. Public Health England (2019). *Prescribed medicines review: report*. [online] GOV.UK. Available at: https://www.gov.uk/government/publications/prescribed-medicines-review-report.

32. Pushkin Industries. (n.d.). *The Happiness Lab with Dr. Laurie Santos*. [online] Available at: https://www.pushkin.fm/podcasts/the-happiness-lab-with-dr-laurie-santos.

33. org. (n.d.). *QRISK3*. [online] Available at: https://qrisk.org.

34. Routley, N. (2021). *A Visual Guide to Human Emotion*. [online] Visual Capitalist. Available at: https://www.visualcapitalist.com/a-visual-guide-to-human-emotion/.

35. Saklayen, M.G. (2018). The Global Epidemic of the Metabolic Syndrome. *Current Hypertension Reports*, [online] 20(2). doi:https://doi.org/10.1007/s11906-018-0812-z.

36. google.co.uk. (n.d.). *Google Scholar.* [online] Available at: https://scholar.google.co.uk/scholar?q=mental+health+study+in+england+2014&hl=en&as_sdt=0&as_vis=1&oi=scholart.

37. Scholes, S. (2017). *Health Survey for England 2016 Physical activity in adults Health Survey for England 2016: Physical activity in adults.* [online] Available at: http://healthsurvey.hscic.gov.uk/media/63730/HSE16-Adult-phy-act.pdf.

38. Simopoulos, A.P., Leaf, A. and Salem, N. (1999). Workshop on the Essentiality of and Recommended Dietary Intakes for Omega-6 and Omega-3 Fatty Acids. *Journal of the American College of Nutrition,* 18(5), pp.487–489. doi:https://doi.org/10.1080/07315724.1999.10718888.

39. Smith, A., Jane, E., Shaw, C., Stansfeld, S., Kamaldeep Bhui and Dhillon, K. (2005). Ethnicity, work characteristics, stress and health.

40. Spector, T. (2019). *You are what you eat – why the future of nutrition is personal.* [online] The Conversation. Available at: https://theconversation.com/you-are-what-you-eat-why-the-future-of-nutrition-is-personal-119477 [Accessed 11 Jul. 2023].

41. Tiedemann, A., Sherrington, C., Bauman, A. and Ding, D. (2023). Supporting physical activity in an ageing world: a call for action. *The Lancet Regional Health - Western Pacific,* 35, p.100546. doi:https://doi.org/10.1016/j.lanwpc.2022.100546.

42. Tutunchi, H., Ebrahimi-Mameghani, M., Ostadrahimi, A. and Asghari-Jafarabadi, M. (2020). What are the optimal cut-off points of anthropometric indices for prediction of overweight and obesity? Predictive validity of waist circumference, waist-to-hip and waist-to-height ratios. *Health Promotion Perspectives,* 10(2), pp.142–147. doi:https://doi.org/10.34172/hpp.2020.23.

43. Viorel Ciorniciuc (2016). *Holmes And Rahe Stress Scale Calculator.* [online] https://www.thecalculator.co. Available at: https://www.thecalculator.co/health/Holmes-And-Rahe-Stress-Scale-Calculator-983.html.

44. (2016). *How to Find Your Tribe.* [online] Available at: https://wanderlust.com/journal/how-to-find-your-tribe/.

45. Wang, Q., Ferreira, D.L.S., Nelson, S.M., Sattar, N., Ala-Korpela, M. and Lawlor, D.A. (2018). Metabolic characterization of menopause: cross-sectional and longitudinal evidence. *BMC Medicine,* 16(1). doi:https://doi.org/10.1186/s12916-018-1008-8.

46. Watson, S. (n.d.). *Harvard Health*. [online] www.health.harvard.edu. Available at: https://www.health.harvard.edu/promotions/sumo/fighting-inflammation.

47. Wild, S., Simiaic, P. and Williams, Z. (2022). Inside Women's Health - BUPA. Available at: https://www.bupa.co.uk/health-information/womens-health.

48. Willett, W., Rockström, J., Loken, B., Springmann, M., Lang, T., Vermeulen, S., Garnett, T., Tilman, D., DeClerck, F., Wood, A., Jonell, M., Clark, M., Gordon, L.J., Fanzo, J., Hawkes, C., Zurayk, R., Rivera, J.A., De Vries, W., Majele Sibanda, L. and Afshin, A. (2019). Food in the Anthropocene: the EAT–Lancet Commission on healthy diets from sustainable food systems. *The Lancet*, [online] 393(10170), pp.447–492. doi:https://doi.org/10.1016/s0140-6736(18)31788-4.

49. World Health Organization (WHO) (2022). *Ageing and health*. [online] World Health Organization. Available at: https://www.who.int/newsroom/fact-sheets/detail/ageing-and-health.

50. health.harvard.edu. (n.d.). *Harvard Health*. [online] Available at: https://www.health.harvard.edu/category/staying-healthy.

51. nogg.org.uk. (n.d.). *Clinical guideline for the prevention and treatment of osteoporosis*. [online] Available at: https://www.nogg.org.uk/full-guideline.

52. psychologytoday.com. (n.d.). *Why Are Balance and Harmony So Vital for Well-being? | Psychology Today*. [online] Available at: https://www.psychologytoday.com/us/blog/finding-light-in-the-darkness/202102/why-are-balance-and-harmony-so-vital-well-being.

The Vanity (Warrior) Project

1. Dass, A. (2021). *The colours we share*. New York, NY: Aperture.

2. Dirty, Sexy History. (2016). *Maybe She's Born With It (Maybe It's Lead!): Powder and Patch in the 17th Century*. [online] Available at: https://dirtysexyhistory.com/2016/10/02/maybe-shes-born-with-it-maybe-its-lead-powder-and-patch-in-the-17th-century/.

3. Franken, A.R. (2019). *New rules for post-patriarchal systems and societies*. [online] Male Feminists Europe. Available at: http://www.male-feminists-europe.org/new-rules-post-patriarchal-systems-societies/.

4. Gomberg, L.E. (2001). What Women in Groups Can Learn from the Goddess. *Women & Therapy*, 23(4), pp.55–69. doi:https://doi.org/10.1300/J015v23n04_05.

5. Hart-Davis, A. (2022). *Home.* [online] The Tweakments Guide. Available at: https://thetweakmentsguide.com.

6. HuffPost UK. (2022). *Aging Gracefully Can Be Scary, But Psychologists Reveal How To Shift Your Narrative.* [online] Available at: https://www.huffingtonpost.co.uk/entry/fear-of-aging_l_627030f5e4b0bc48f57e5293.

7. Johns Hopkins Medicine (2021). *9 Benefits of Yoga.* [online] www.hopkinsmedicine.org. Available at: https://www.hopkinsmedicine.org/health/wellness-and-prevention/9-benefits-of-yoga.

8. Julie Hewett LA / Hue Cosmetics Inc. (2016). *The History WHY Women Wear Lipstick.* [online] Available at: https://www.juliehewettla.com/en-gb/blogs/blog/why-do-women-wear-lipstick.

9. Kearney-Cooke, A. and Tieger, D. (2015). Body Image Disturbance and the Development of Eating Disorders. *The Wiley Handbook of Eating Disorders*, pp.283–296. doi:https://doi.org/10.1002/9781118574089.ch22.

10. Maltz, M. and Powers, M. (2010). *Psycho-cybernetics : a new way to get more living out of life.* Chatsworth, Calif.: Wilshire Book Co.

11. com. (2017). *6 Modern Societies Where Women Rule.* [online] Available at: https://www.mentalfloss.com/article/31274/6-modern-societies-where-women-literally-rule.

12. Pagliarini, M.A. (1999). The Pure American Woman and the Wicked Catholic Priest: An Analysis of Anti-Catholic Literature in Antebellum America. *Religion and American Culture: A Journal of Interpretation*, [online] 9(1), pp.97–128. doi:https://doi.org/10.2307/1123928.

13. Riji, H.M. (2006). Beauty Or Health? A Personal View. *Malaysian Family Physician : the Official Journal of the Academy of Family Physicians of Malaysia*, [online] 1(1), pp.42–44. Available at: https://www.ncbi.nlm.nih.gov/pmc/articles/PMC4797041/.

14. Robinson-Moore, C.L. (2008). Beauty Standards Reflect Eurocentric Paradigms-So What? Skin Color, Identity, and Black Female Beauty. 4(1), p.66.

15. Ruiz, M. (2016). *The Geography of Beauty: Beauty standards across the globe.* [online] Project Vanity. Available at: http://www.projectvanity.com/projectvanity/beauty-standards-across-the-globe.

16. Stang, S.M. (2021). Maiden, Mother, and Crone: Abject Female Monstrosity in Roleplaying Games. *ca.* [online] doi:http://hdl.handle.net/10315/38644.

17. Van Edwards, V. (2016). *Beauty Standards: See How Body Types Change Through History.* [online] Science of People. Available at: https://www.scienceofpeople.com/beautystandards/#:~:text=Beauty%20in%20the%201920s%20featured.

18. Walton, G. (2014). *Ideas of Female Beauty in the 1700 and 1800s.* [online] Geri Walton. Available at: https://www.geriwalton.com/ideas-of-female-beauty-in-1700-and-1800s/.

19. psychologytoday.com. (n.d.). *Appreciating the Difference Between Pride and Vanity | Psychology Today United Kingdom.* [online] Available at: https://www.psychologytoday.com/gb/blog/the-art-and-science-aging-well/201701/appreciating-the-difference-between-pride-and-vanity.

Book Club Questions

Each of the women is at a crossroads. They have to make wise decisions for their future. Think of each chapter and answer these questions:

1. All six women in their life stories wear masks of some description, real or symbolic. Which masks can be attributed to each character?
2. Think of each character and discuss what decisions they *should* make going forward?
3. Now that you've been party to their backstories and habits, and based on the balance of probabilities, what decisions are they more likely to make?
4. How does their stage of menopause impact their life currently, and which podcast will they need to revisit?
5. What's the significance of the challenges and obstacles in the Vanity Project?
6. Did you align the Queens with their real life characters? If so, can you pin the suitable tweakments on the right queen?

A final thought. Having read the book and knowing these characters intimately, now begin to look around—at every train station, at work, or at every social gathering. Can you spot them? Which one are you? Or are you a blend?

Rules of the game - Risk to Reward

BTM: In summary, **Risk2Reward®** the game, has been stacked with specific and relevant events, emotions, hazards, and the risks associated with middle-aged women 40-60 years. It is a work of fiction. Creative or artistic licence has allowed us to play devil's advocate with how we have selected the cards, the emotional responses, and the behavioural hazards. It was never going to be a game of chance!

BTM: RISK2REWARD®

Level One: Create the Avatar
Every player will need an avatar. You can play with your metrics or make it up.
Age, BMI, Waist-Hip Ratio, existing health conditions etc

Level Two: Map your Risk Zone
You start the game at age forty on the Health Risk Zone using:
1) your BMI and
2) your Waist-Hip ratio
3) Existing Health Conditions

Collectively these represent your statistical health risk.

Zones are shades of Green, Yellow, Amber and Red, which indicates the risk spectrum from No, Low, Medium to High. Red Zone indicates chronic stress and/or chronic illness and belongs to the medical professionals.

The positions on the board are determined by throwing three dice.
 Dice One advances the years.
Dice Two shows the number of Life Events (LE), which you select at random.
Dice Three gives you a choice of Behavioural Hazards (BH) with their Associated Risks attached (AR). For the readers' clarity, in the diagram we have numbered the behavioural hazard with its corresponding numbered risk.

Emotional Response Cards
When Life Event cards are in play, you choose which Emotional Response (ER) cards are suitable. These cards carry their own health risk levels, meaning that the same Emotional Response card can represent a different health risks: No, Low, Medium, High. This places them in the appropriate zone.

Wild cards represent unexpected events, calamities, hazards and responses. High-Risk Wild cards change the direction of play and can potentially place you in the Red Zone.

Routine health checks occur at designated points, and the results determine the direction of travel across the zones.

The outcome of a player's choice to 'Walk Tall' into a LOW-RISK Zone or 'Stumble Fall' into a HIGH-RISK Zone will only be revealed in the next move.

The game will unfold as players progress.

Risk to Reward - Part 1

BTM: RISK2REWARD®

Level Three: What is the Rewards Model?

It is a diagnostic tool that is more holistic than just using BMI as the main driver for health. We all know that what we are thinking and feeling impacts our choices of eating and moving, which further affects our level of connecting to restore our spirit.

Control - indicator measures Feeling and Thinking.
Health - indicator measures Nutrition and Movement.
Connect - indicator measures Self-esteem and Network (points of contact)

The markers combine to place you in health risk zones:
Outer zones represent no-to-low health risks; You're REWARDING yourself!
Inner zones represent alarm, with less favourable results and higher health risks.
Red zone or high stress zone, as we already know, means seek professional help!

Collectively with algorithms in place, and the completion of levels one and two, this model will also produce a score that determines how you use the six simple rewards across all domains.

The three domains are:
Between **Control** and **Health** is PSYCHOLOGICAL **(Mind)**.
Between **Health** and **Connect** is PHYSICAL **(Body)**.
Between **Connect** and **Control** are RELATIONSHIPS, SOCIAL & CULTURAL **(Spirit)**.

The user primarily drives this level, with the prospect of interfacing with other wellbeing data sources and medical biomarkers to achieve a more accurate result.

When inputted, results of expert investigations or medical biomarkers will always override the outcomes presented here. Fundamentally, the user's perspective and narrative will guide an exploration into all aspects of life that can impact your overall health: life events, emotional responses, stress management, and connectivity.

This model is designed to empower the user by producing a personal and meaningful action plan to achieve the relevant six simple rewards.

Risk to Reward - Part 2

ACKNOWLEDGEMENTS

What a thrilling ride this has been for both of us and we didn't do it alone.

What started with data collection, instinct and certainty was met with suggestions from a few who truly listened to what we were aiming to achieve.

It has taken us on quite a journey of discovery. Our writing journey began around a kitchen table with a flipchart and our insatiable curiosity and very quickly this book was mapped out in an afternoon and began to morph into acquiring a much wider brief. One that encompasses every woman in mid life with its complexity and multiple layers: ageing, life events and the hormonal shift.

Heartfelt thanks go to Bradley Theodore, artist and listener extraordinaire, who sees into the bare bones of people. Nicola Rossi for sharing a realistic and determined view of publishing. James Bannon for his frank kindness in telling us just how it is. Marie Morley for guiding where to try and reach out. We took all your recommendations seriously.

Of course, words cannot express our love for our family and friends. We are aware how obsessed and consumed we have been. Your support and patience has been unwavering. Special love and acknowledgement to James Crichton; couldn't have done this without your belief and commitment. The chocolate biscuits are on us.

We take a bow to the strong female writers before us who set the tone for expressing courage in middle age. We woke up to the fact that it's the 21st Century and now is not the time to be coy; it's time to get real.

A huge thank you to those who were willing to freely give their time to review our earlier manuscripts: James Bannon, Lara Berni-Klerk, Dr Alice Chiswick, Jeanie Civil, James Crichton, Michelle Doyle, Ross Davidson; Juliette Every, Kerry McNally, and Vicki Rayment. We have taken on board all your valuable and considered feedback.

A salute to sculptor, Matt Buckley with the cover image (courtesy of justsculptures.com.) Everyone loves the cover!

Not forgetting Rebecca Crichton for her creative input and time. Patience is one of your many virtues.

Lastly, to our Mothers and Mothers-in-law, you set the bar so very high. We love and celebrate you.

ABOUT THE AUTHORS

Susanne Every

Is an international development consultant working across all business sectors and has coached and mentored executives for decades. She's creative and wildly curious. Whilst being a devoted mother of four, in her spare time she designed, project-managed and built the family home. Now delighted to be in a partnership with a new focus. She's a woeful golfer but an excellent spoiler of dogs. The family moved from London 20 years ago to live in the English countryside. The dogs continue to be spoiled and her golfing abilities remain a challenge.

Deidre Crichton

Is now a published author and partner in an exciting new venture. An accountant by profession, she has lived and worked in Johannesburg, Munich, Dubai and now England. Her project management experience in financial and hospitality software, including systems architecture has been across various industries. She's also a creative type although balanced with a continuous desire for self-improvement and altruism. She's especially family oriented, is a decent golfer and has had a lifelong obsession with dogs.

Milton Keynes UK
Ingram Content Group UK Ltd.
UKHW022115021023
429810UK00012B/85